Giggling Dr. Green

Yael Shany

Saving our children for our planet

Giggling Dr. Green

Disclaimer

(The legal stuff I have to say, because we live in a litigious society.)

The information provided in this book is not to be considered medical advice. Readers are encouraged to obtain help from doctors and other licensed medical practitioners, as well as their services and recommendations.

Please note that none of the parties involved in the writing and producing of this book, including but not limited to the author, publisher, editor, designer, and incidental contributors to the creation of this book, are medically trained professionals.

Since this book, Giggling Dr. Green, is a health and wellness enhancing guideline and suggestions book and NOT a medical advice or prescription book by any means, it has not and will not be granted FDA approval as a medical book.

Please note that the authors as well as the publisher of this book have used their freedom of speech to express their own personal views, experiences and philosophy, and assume absolutely no responsibility for any health problem, deterioration or adverse results that may affect the reader or any party who decides to follow these guidelines. Personal decisions to follow any suggestions found in this book, with or without reactions or results, positive or negative are solely on the individual's own responsibility and said individuals will never be able to bring forth any claims against the author or anybody who took part in the creation of this book.

If you think you are suffering from a serious medical condition, see your doctor. Do not attempt to self-diagnose. Tell your doctor if you are taking homeopathic remedies, and what they consist of. You should never disregard medical advice or delay in seeking it because of something you have read in this book.

Homeopathy is considered (in our era) an alternative approach to health and wellness and is not a substitute for medical treatment. Any information, education, remedies, and/or therapies suggested in this book do not include any form of medical diagnosis, and all therapies, remedies, treatments, exercises, or

Giggling Dr. Green

diet changes should be undertaken only under the supervision of a properly trained health care professional.

If you think you may have a medical emergency,

Giggling Dr. Green

Dedication

I thank Aki for saying "If this book will save just one child in the world, it is worth your work".

Maayan, thank you for supporting me on this mission writing Giggling Dr. Green through our fruitful conversations, even when you were so tired you could barely talk anymore. Maayan, you are a role model for me and many other mothers. Thank you for your contribution and deep devoted love. Maayan, thank you for supporting me on this mission writing Giggling Dr. Green through our fruitful conversations, even when you were so tired you could barely talk anymore. Maayan, you are a role model for me and many other mothers. Thank you for your contribution and deep devoted love.

The idea to put my thoughts, opinions and some of my vast experience I have accumulated all these years was yours. Shay, you have been so often my mentor and support, my inspiration and though my son, yet my great teacher. Thank you for all you have done for me in all these years since I have had you.

Tal, as my youngest son you have been teaching me the wisdom of raising a son who was born with more challenges than your siblings, yet your achievements reminded me that everything is possible under the sun. You inspired me throughout your life to - never give up optimism, the little child in me and laughter. Thank you for everything in you that helped and contributed to me and the world through this book,

Omrie you have always been my young soulmate and you Edoh and Nadav, my dear grandsons. Thank you for your permission to show you to the world and tell the world about you. I am proud of you.

Alex, you are my youngest grandson, my heart and my soul. Your beautiful personality is the light on my path to optimism, kindness and compassion.

To all of you who taught me all I know, thanks for helping all the children who may, so help me God, benefit and heal through the ideas and guidance offered in this book. I pray for this book to save the lives of as many precious children in the world as possible.

Giggling Dr. Green

May this book help to change the world into a better, safer and healthier place for us and future generations to come. I hope that Giggling Dr. Green will contribute to saving our planet for our children and our children for our planet.

Thank you, dear Johnny, for giving me the opportunity to help you the best I possibly could. Special thanks to you Johnny for having the courage and the big smile to see the beauty in the world and teaching me humbleness as well as the infinite powers of nature. You are my light and will always stay in my heart.

Yael

September 2018 (the date was changed in order to include Alex

Giggling Dr. Green

Prologue

Dear Johnny

You came to me through Divine Powers to assist me in the writing of this book.
You have come to me, so that I can do the speaking for you. The entire world
must know your story and I will tell you it. Together we will help parents save
their children from experiencing the despair, agony, sadness and pain you
endure daily.

When you first came to me, I thought that although you were yet another
casualty of the mandatory vaccinations policy in America (as well as all the other
medically advanced countries), your body would probably be able to recover, and
you would be able to resume a normal child's life. I was so terribly wrong. It was
not only the vaccinations that harmed your small body so seriously; it was the
medications they had forced you into to control the reactions to the devastating
side effects of the vaccinations. Vaccinations deemed essential, and therefore
given by rote, in the 'modern and medically advanced' U.S.A. The medication
prescribed to 'tidy up' the seizures you had after each vaccination was
Phenobarbital, which is indicated in the use of 'severe mental disorders and
multiple-personality illnesses. You, an infant, were given a barbiturate, which
depressed the activity of your brain and nervous system. The side effects of
Phenobarbital can include over excitement, irritability, aggression, depression, or
confusion, particularly in children. If overdosed, what could happen? "Symptoms
of a Phenobarbital overdose include difficulty breathing, back and forth
movements of the eyes, the

appearance of being drunk, rapid heartbeat, low body temperature, heavy
sedation, coma, and death."

Your parents had none of this explained to them before they allowed it to
be given to you when you were just 2 years old. When you first came to me, you
were 14 months old, yet, stuck in the developmental stage of a 2-month-old. Your
parents had been told, "There was nothing they could do to help you", by the very
doctors who set you on this path of pain and anguish.

Johnny, I believe you know how every soul has a purpose on this planet. I
also believe you understand that every soul chooses their body and the parents to
be born to, in order to complete this "mission" on our planet. You chose to
sacrifice your childhood in order to be a silent voice crying in the wilderness.

Giggling Dr. Green

Your deafening silence forces us to listen and examine the changes that we must affect.

Your silent struggle spoke volumes into my heart, and your affliction became my burden. I cannot close my eyes to rest and not see the injustice that has so deeply injured you, and so many other infants and children by the mainstream medicine machine. God blessed you with parents who are determined never to rest until you improve. Their journey is as long as your life. Nevertheless, you are also so brave and determined that I pray to the Universe, and God, that your cry will help all those other children who must be saved, lest they join you in your torment.

Johnny, you are my inspiration to write this book and face all the controversy I expect to face. Are you able to understand how strong and forceful true justice is in America? Yet, stronger and bigger, still, is the Universal Justice for children. Children are born innocent. They come to this world with no thoughts, opinions, expectations, prejudices or judgments. Children come to this planet with one very strong asset, an innate trust in goodness and love. You came to our *world with the very same asset. I pray that you in your little* world still hold on to it and never lose it. Because, thanks to people like you, eventually things will change. The greed of the pharmaceutical companies must stop at a certain point. Those unfortunate people, who own the pharmaceutical companies, must not enjoy the hope of love and goodness, as you do. Therefore, I would like you to be able, if you can, to forgive them. I am certain they did not intentionally harm you or wish upon you the irreversible damage that their products caused. They just felt the dark fear of poverty. They are scared to death of not having enough. Johnny, you are still not familiar with that overwhelming fear. It has the power to destroy lives, and it has, so many times. This fear of not having enough provokes these pitiable, pathetic people to produce medications that they know very well are harmful and damaging to children, and yet, the medicines supply them with the money they need so badly to quiet their fears. They are probably very weak and unhappy people. Though they may have a seat in Congress, which makes them feel very important, they are actually scared to death of their own products. They know that when they get sick, the doctors will serve them the same medications they know kill all the others, mainly the young, innocent, loving children. These people are certainly aware of the power of Karma. Oh Johnny, do they pray that the Universe will not turn the wheel and manifest the law of 'what goes around comes around' towards them. Even though you are so young and suffer an extremely compromised childhood and future because of their cowardice, I hope you are able to forgive them. They, after all, have to live with their conscience, getting up every morning to a new day of haunting thoughts, "What I create, that

Giggling Dr. Green

makes me so wealthy and lets me live in this extravagant mansion, harms and even kills children like Johnny every day. How will my Karma be? When will I have to pay for my reckless, devastating greed? I am even afraid to look into the mirror and see what a monster I have become. Do I really need that much money? Certainly not. However, I am too frightened to admit that even to myself. If you rose up and called me a murderer for the children I have helped to massacre, through my lack of knowledge or courage, I would not be surprised. One day the truth will be unveiled. I am scared that my children and grandchildren will have to suffer the same ramifications as Johnny has.

You see Johnny, this is the reason for this book. We are compelled to let all the parents in America, and the rest of the 'medically advanced' world of mandatory childhood vaccinations, know what must save their children from the same destiny you suffer daily. It will be hard to get everything on paper because, as you know, there are such horrifically sad stories that we risk the chance people will not be able to believe them. However, Johnny, we must try. I know that this is the full purpose of our paths crossing. Your presence in my life opened a floodgate of memories of all the children whose lives I have tried to save after the medical establishment's mandatory, monstrous rules and regulations had compromised their health. Even now, their lawyers are trying to pass a law to quiet people like me, who are fighting for you and all of your brothers and sisters. We have witnessed the damage in far too many children, because they pass laws allowing the continuation of this barbaric practice. Continuing to kill your pals and kill the life force in those who are still alive, but do not even know how to chew their food, at the age of five, all because of mandatory vaccinations and medications. The petitions against these unconscionable mandates are out, and the battles we must win are at hand.

Dear Johnny, thank God you are not aware of how many children will be handicapped in your generation alone and what the face of our nation will be like in 20 years. Everything will have to change. Businesspeople will have to work in different environments because 60-80 percent will be ADD, ADHD, Autistic, Obese, Diabetic, and all the other horrible results of the vaccinations. They are the lucky ones who are alive and able to be halfway functional. The others will be in nursing centers and will have to receive complete care their entire lives. Then there are those who are much less fortunate, who simply died on their way to start a new life of hope, goodness, and love their parents intended them to.

Dear Johnny, we all know the truth. However, is the world ready to serve and support the damage the government supports to create? The standards will have to change. Drivers will have to undergo different guidelines, and perhaps cars

Giggling Dr. Green

will have to undergo adjustments to the new human standards. Like the furniture making industry has to adjust and design super-sized chairs and beds, like the aircraft engineers have to redesign the seat sizes for the extra big people the pharmaceutical companies gradually helped to create. So will everything else have to adjust. Normal healthy children, whose parents decide to 'break the law' and have their kids not vaccinated turn suddenly to be the minority. These 'normal' kids will become abnormal like for example, our grandkids, will require check-ups to determine if everything is alright with them. My own blood work results were under suspicion, because I have not been taking any medications at my age. So, my dear sweet Johnny, do you understand now what your soul came into this body for? To compel me to communicate the message your heart cries out.

Love   Yael

Giggling Dr. Green

" **To all parents** and grandparents, pharmaceutical company owners, members of Congress and media owners, as well as the medical community, Food manufacturers, Toys manufacturers, and all of you who should rethink the purpose of each one of us on this planet.

Yael has known me for the past 2 1/2 years. I know her hands, her voice and her loving eyes. I cannot talk to her because I am unable to speak more than just 'oh' 'bell' and make a kissing sound. Nevertheless, I hear Yael's conversations with my mother. She is doing her best to help me walk, talk, chew my food, focus my eyes, hold my head up, grow and be healthy.

Please, read this book and help your children grow up healthy, functional and most of all, let them giggle as only children can. If you will listen to Yael you will actually be listening to thousands of children like me who are here to warn you: 'Do not let them kill us'. Please stop the senseless slaughter of our future. Please, help these pharmaceutical company owners to make as much money as they could possibly desire without harming and killing us children. There is so much money out there, they can have it all, just, please, let us live and build a strong new generation of normal healthy people. We want to be fully functioning citizens, who are positive factors in the building and development of our wonderful country. We long to be able to contribute to our great nation, and not just require constant handling by others, feeding us, changing us, walking us and carrying us about in our damaged bodies, our personal prisons. We deserve it. We have the right to live. We did not choose to be a burden on our parents and society. Please, listen and fight for us.

With love, hope, and goodness,

Johnny".

Chapter One
My mission

For well over 60 years, I have been completely devoted to fighting for children like Johnny, for their health, safety and well-being. I have a personal collection of far too many sad stories, some of which I share with you in this book. Thankfully, however, I also have some wonderful victories to inspire you. My lifelong goal has been to help all people, children and adults, find the light at the end of the health tunnel. In our generation, that light must shine brightly for the little babies and the children. I truly regret having to say that, but they are the most innocent victims of the Medical Establishment Greed Agenda (MEGA), and at the same time they are the least able to defend themselves. Their misguided parents are so afraid to go against the rules and regulations, and most still live in the darkness of the third millennium with their belief in the 'good intentions of the medical community' that every baby born is a potential victim of the MEGA force. New babies will suffer through vaccinations and may then begin a lifelong struggle with criminally imposed handicaps and ill health. If this baby is very lucky, she or he will make it, yet the number of the less fortunate is increasing. Even as I write this there is a debate on Israeli TV about the various childhood vaccinations and they counted 25 different diseases inoculated into these newborn innocent victims, and in the US, they mount to 39 already. (06/06/07)

My intention in this book is not to advocate the absolute shut down of all mainstream medicine. Certainly, many parts of mainstream medicine have absolute value. My fight is against the unnecessary medication of children, of ruthless vaccinations, even though it is avoidable in our country today. I fight against the 'Dr. God syndrome' that decrees only the prescribed medications; surgery and radiation methods will be used. When a mainstream doctor speaks about PEMF, (Pulsed Electromagnetic Field Therapy), Reflexology, or Reiki, most doctors will say, "That is nothing but nonsense" or "bewitchery". I must fight against the undemocratic Congressional bill that prohibits any alternative medicine or methods other than those offered under the authority of a Medical Doctor. These MDs never learned anything about natural health and the immune system's miraculous self-healing mechanism. So, why is it that a citizen in a democratic country may not choose what medical path is right for him? Why allow American citizens to suffer from the MD's ignorance? Who died and declared the Congress, FDA and AMA to be God Almighty, to allow or prohibit what each one of us can choose to do with our own health? In all but truly all, other countries and continents around the world are a simple given. Every person can make these basic, natural choices even if admitted to a hospital. When I just started my studies, I was happy to learn that in every hospital in Europe, you could choose which medical applications you prefer. I suppose many of us, in the Complementary Medical practitioner's community, will have to 'pay a little visit to jail' before this miraculous right is granted to the US citizens.

When I first moved to the US, I was under the illusion that this huge and beautiful country would also be the most culturally, scientifically and democratic advanced country in the world. Up until the point when I was asked for the first but not last time, "What is Homeopathy?" I was shocked later on to learn how the Pharmaceutical Establishment and the FDA and AMA, keep so much vital knowledge and access to it from their citizens who have a legitimate right and need to the information they keep so closely guarded. I discovered that the 'Golden Rule', meaning 'Whoever has the most gold, rules', governs this country. The MEGA Force and their coalition of money first groups of medicine and medical instrument industry affiliates care only for their wallets, for which they are willing to sacrifice even their own children. (One of the doctor's wives asked me, "Aren't you scared to be killed for your thoughts?")

Each day I become even more astonished. Yes, I am determined to bring out all my thoughts and conclusions, my experience and good advice to all those who may choose to learn and know about it. Even if I am forced to leave this beautiful, yet somewhat corrupt country, the value of truth will be well worth it. People will be able to get the book from other countries if America bans it.

I will still try to do my best to save as many innocent children as I can. In the name of Johnny.

If you find my ideas are too extreme for you and that it is not the way you would like to proceed with your own children, I completely understand. This book is not intended to be a 'cure all ', and not even an instruction book. However, everyone who has chosen to try my suggestions, for them or for their children, has experienced rapid and noticeable improvement in their overall health. Since very little can be declared absolutely, and there are as many different ways and approaches to health as there are different personalities, all I want is to introduce my readers to the summary of 53 years' experience in complementary and true medicine.

I pray that our next generations will be healthier than the youngsters of today, and will be able to form a better, more positive future nation than it is today. The magic of synchronicity is that, as I am working on this book, all over the TV and radio stations worldwide, from many different sources, the message is the same, "We must provide better conditions for the children to grow up healthier. After all, our true success is not in the title our child may hold some day, but the quality of life, health, and happiness she or he has.

Over the counter misleading solutions

Walking through the grocery superstores here in the US is a staggering experience for most first timers. The abundance and variety is amazing. However, besides all the wonderful food displays you can find as many medications as you like. That was the real eye opener for me; I could not believe it when I walked through the pharmacy department and found medications that only a doctor's prescription should provide. My first reaction was "How liberal", yet, as I continued to examine the array of drugs so readily available, I came to consider it as dangerous and highly recommend banning that level of accessibility of those. After all there is not even one harmless and side effects-free medication.

Far worse is that everyone can purchase any medication on a supermarket or even gas station display. How useless is it to try and help the drug addicts and arrest the drug peddlers, if drugs are so openly at reach everywhere. We raise our children to believe instant relief is available for every discomfort, yet, who supervises the proper use and dosages? Who are the true criminals in the real drug peddlers here?

The pharmaceutical company's managers and the government lawmakers; those are the biggest drug pushers and enablers in the US. The reality is that the law fights the victims of the medical establishment. The law should point the finger at the real source of this problem, where it begins - with the lawmakers. If the pharmaceutical companies did not have free reign to display those huge quantities of drugs so openly, the public would not expect a quick and easy answer to every health concern. It would change the whole war against drugs immediately.

Giggling Dr. Green

Following the massive money trail, we discover the government knows very well the MEGA Force will never allow all the removal of the so-called over-the-counter drugs from the public's access, since it amounts to billions of dollars a year in revenue. Look around and see how much misery you are around; how many people are victims of the very medicine that was supposed to be the answer to their pain and suffering.

Now let us consider our children; I am certainly not suggesting they not be offered relief for their illnesses and pain; we absolutely must support and comfort them. My suggestion is always to try natural and harmless methods of pain relief before reaching for the dangerous and damaging side effects causing drugs. I advocate allowing fever to run its course without suppressing it with medications. A cool wet cloth, applied to the child that has a fever, will bring comfort, while still supporting the immune system in its efforts towards natural healing. When we suppress the fever, we may cause many devastating and long-lasting side effects, for instance; the body will stop fighting for its own health because we have "unarmed" it and quieted its means to do so. Fever is the best indicator for imbalance and the best tool to restore good health.

The MEGA Force labels fever with various names, such as flu, virus, inflammation, infection etc. and with its misleading propaganda advocates fighting it by heavy medications. In nature it is merely indicating an imbalance in the body, and the root cause must be discovered. For example, when the acidity level rises even a small amount, the cells start to lack oxygen, creating the proper foundation for different protein chains to develop. That is a threat to healthy cells, and the natural balance is off. The white blood cells and the lymphatic system will then fight the fever and imbalance, the natural way. In the natural health arena, we recognize it as a healthy process, simply a natural reaction of a healthy and normal organism to protect the body and re-establish balance. This is the reason for fever, it is the natural indication that the immune system is fighting for the body's health. If we take the initiative and use drugs to stop the fever, we actually disarm the body, enabling the foreign proteins to continue to thrive with nothing to hinder them, this way we have effectively disabled the immune system.

The very same truth applies to skin rashes, diarrhea, headaches, hives, heartburn, nausea etc.; they all are a natural way of the body to help the organs transport and expel toxins out of the body. We all grew up learning to keep our bodies clean; wouldn't this be true for the inside as well as the outside? We certainly understand never tolerate invaders in our homes, so shouldn't we guard our bodies as well? We must not allow the physicians to silence our child's alarm system, effectively disarming their natural ability to stop the harmful invaders.

Giggling Dr. Green

Why do we let them inhibit our child's natural self-defense mechanism to do the job naturally?

Why do we allow the pharmaceutical companies to brainwash us with their misleading and damaging panic? Every day, morning to night, while watching TV, we are allowing them to spoon feed us with the MEGA Force's newest moneymaker, new medication. It is no secret that these commercials help turn big profits, but we do not have to allow that brainwashing into our homes. If we have a sleeping disorder and see on TV how quick and easy it is to pop a pill to wake rested and refreshed in the morning, we do not question the claims, or side effects, because the commercial producers know exactly how to numb our judgment, while lining their own guilty pockets. How many people will be permanently damaged prior to the announcement of the next major drug recall? How many victims will never wake up again after taking that magic pill?

I vividly recall the terrible results so many babies endured because their mothers took Thalidomide medication while pregnant. Children were born with deformed limbs or none at all. Do you remember how many malformed children were born after the Desert Storm War? Extensive evidence supported the belief that the massive vaccinations their deployed parents received were at the root of that horrible after-effect; however, the government hushed it up very quickly. Again, following the money trail we discover the pharmaceutical companies made a lot of money during and directly after that war.

On the other hand, have you ever seen any commercial for alternative, natural medicine or methods? Have you ever seen the mainstream media disclose research results for homeopathic medicine? Or about any harmful side effects from using fresh lemon, cool wet cloth or a homeopathic remedy? I have not, and the argument I always receive is, "Your medicine is not scientifically proven, whereas mainstream medicine is". True? No. All natural healing means have been scientifically proven.

In 1995 I happened to listen to an interview on WLRN in which scientists revealed a decades old secret. They disclosed the truth behind the vaccines, however these facts never showed up on the TV commercials when they advertise flu shots, for example. I was delighted to hear the truth behind the faulty myth 'miraculous difference' vaccinations have made in the present health conditions, however, for economic and commercial reasons, the truth and warnings regarding the vaccinations have never reached the vast public. I will get to that subject in more detail in the chapter of vaccines.

Giggling Dr. Green

I like to encourage all parents, please be attentive to the inner voice that guides you before administering any medication. Always keep in mind how every medication has harmful side effects and suppresses important vital functions that should not be ignored. Every medication will require a counter medication to 'undo' the damage of the previous one. Every medication has the potential to rob your child's body of its natural given skills to defend it and grow up, balanced, normal, healthy and strong.

Notice:

For every ailment there is an answer. Unlike the mainstream answer of suppression and damage, the natural way is supporting and healing for a strong, stable and consistent health and well-being. Ask and you shall receive; seek a good therapist, natural healer or do the research yourself with all the vast available information. The applications are natural, simple, and very inexpensive; everyone can do it. Clear your thoughts of all the commercials you have been listening to all these years, and the fears they have implanted in your heart. Remember, humankind has existed for many more centuries than the pharmaceutical industry, and in spite not having all the over-the-counter drugs to fix every ailment.

Prevention

As a child, Tad was not disciplined enough to thoroughly brush his teeth every day, or instead, chew on hard fresh fruits and vegetables. The amount of sugar-laden food he consumed was amazing. Tad grew up with these same bad habits. By the age of 30, he started to pay for his poor oral hygiene habits and his gums became a very troubling source of poor health. Anyone could see the compromised state of Tad's health by the offensive breath, color, and condition of his teeth and gums. Tad's parents should have trained him to keep his mouth clean by regular brushing and should have been supervised for his compliance. It is not just the teeth affected; the gums also suffer from poor oral care. (I highly recommend avoiding any commercial toothpaste).

When we eat raw foods like apples and carrots, the biting and chewing required actually clean the teeth and massage the gums. Therefore, whenever we serve our child raw fruits and vegetables we contribute to their health. Does this seem too simple to you to be true? Juices released during active chewing of fresh fruit naturally destroy bacteria and fungus in the inner soft tissues of the mouth for lack of those juices and chewing. Eating cooked food actually supports the harmful bacteria and fungus growing in our mouths, because it does not build the same active juices the raw fruit and vegetables do. The cooked food leaves plenty of residues behind. When serving cooked food in one bowl, and raw vegetables in the second bowl, after both bowls had been emptied, the difference in the residue can clearly be seen. The PH environment we want in our mouth is alkaline, which the raw food helps to create, unlike the cooked food that creates a very acidic environment. The ideal fertile ground for bacteria is an acidic environment and for good health, we need an alkaline environment.

The problem with unhealthy teeth and gums is not only the unpleasant appearance and odor. Keep in mind that the blood circulation that runs through our mouth runs through our entire body. Left to grow, unhealthy bacteria and fungus in our mouths will compromise the natural, healthy balance throughout the whole body. Inflamed gums and decayed teeth will have an unhealthy impact on the kidney, liver and heart just like any other infection in the body would.

Sadly, Tad will need to have his teeth removed because of the amount of damage that accumulated. Had his parents been more aware of preventive medicine, he would be much healthier today, and his teeth would not have deteriorated. We always need to see the complete picture of health for our children. Do not approach oral health as in allopathic medicine, treating all organs, different systems and diseases as separate. It is all one big, complex and magnificent orchestra that has to play together in harmony. This is true good health, and preventive medicine is our number one responsibility.

Teeth are made of very important minerals and tissues the body produces. However, when you teach your child to brush the teeth after each meal, make sure you do not fall into the trap of the commercial lies, based on misinformation from the FDA regarding fluoride use. Fluoride is not necessary for healthy teeth; it is a dangerous, chemical poison, sheer industrial waste. For no better way to dispose of it, fluoride winds up in our drinking water and dental hygiene products. Make sure to keep your child fluoride free and avoid the ruthless disregard for our health in this product. It is another government that endorsed and accepted crime that no one seems to care about correcting. Please, only purchase toothpaste that clearly states, "Fluoride free". For more information about fluoride Google, it on the internet and search for information about this poisonous, routinely added element in our children's toothpaste, you will be horrified. Simply because they have no other way to market this industrial waste, our children are subject to its effects. Even when writing these words, I cannot believe that awful truth.

The other aspect of oral health and disease prevention is curtailing candy and dessert consumption as well as overly cooked and processed food. Even meat and dairy products can attack the health of teeth and gums. One reason is the PH

Giggling Dr. Green

balance that I mentioned previously. You know very well when you have a pet
how the vet insists on having its teeth cleaned regularly. This is necessary for
domestic animals because we supply them with a diet of food that is processed and
filled with anything but natural food. They do not have to "struggle" and chew, as
wild animals must. These foods deteriorate the pet's gums and teeth just as the
average American diet does our gums and teeth. Much like building and
maintaining our bone density through lifting and resistance, so are our teeth and
gums. They too need the frequent resistance against hard to chew, fresh foods,
which cause friction on the teeth and gums. Over-cooked, processed, artificial,
sugar laden foods help create an ideal environment for aggressive and damaging
bacteria to thrive.

Fruit juices, soda, etc. add significantly to those same damaging
conditions. I suggest helping children maintain good health and prevent any health
problems by serving fresh, unprocessed foods; no meat, poultry or fish are
necessary for them to thrive. Neither are they necessary for adults, but this book
deals with children's health and well-being in a natural and preventative way.

Another very misleading, dangerous and very harmful myth is that
children need dairy for their bones and teeth. This is as far from the truth as the
east is from the west. The truth is that the dairy industry propaganda for their
products and monetary gains is all it is. There is not even one drop of truth in that
old dairy myth. Almond's milk has significantly more digestible calcium than any
dairy product, and the same can be said for sesame seed milk, rice milk, soy milk,
many other seed derived products, and of course mother's milk. Consider the
overwhelming differences when our children consume almond products and vegan
milk; they do not have the ear infections, skin irritations and colds children get
when served dairy products. Would you believe that dairy products are bad for
your children's teeth and gums? Well, they certainly are. The reasons are the same
as I have mentioned before, regarding the plaque they leave on the teeth, the
acidity, and the fertile ground for bacteria to thrive. I will address the damage to
our kidneys and immune system in other chapters. Pour a glass of milk and empty
it after an hour. You can see the film on the glass walls left, reminding you that in
this glass was milk. This same film clogs the arteries. Try to leave it out in the sun
for 6 hours and then smell it. This is what happens to the milk in your child's
mouth and intestines.

Dental hygiene prevents disease

You can raise your child as far away from conventional dentistry as you like by avoiding those foods and preventing damage. They do not tell you to avoid serving all these damaging foods, and add in the healthy foods. That information would not be good for business. Children do not have to accumulate plague, and can therefore avoid deep dental scraping, as they do to pets. It is simple, easy and will keep your child in excellent oral health, and yet not exclusively the mouth, but the whole body will benefit. Remember: the same plaque that accumulates on the teeth later will accumulate in the blood vessels. This is when the good doctor steps in and inserts stents, balloons, artificial arteries, bypasses, cardiac medications, heart transplants, kidney transplants etc. to correct the failing health. We can raise our children to be strong and healthy, by making them aware of natural health maintenance and prevention of disease. It is so simple, does not cost any extra, and preserves quality of health and life.

All those suggestions are relevant for the digestive system as well. If we really desire to help our child to prevent disease, every meal should start with fresh juicy fruit or fresh vegetables. We must remove syrup, cereal with milk, eggs, peanut butter on white bread sandwiches, processed meat and any other food that is overcooked and sugar laden from our children's diets. Breakfast must not start with warm cocoa and marshmallows, or with any canned fruit juice product. Only with fresh apple, grapefruit, berries, cherries, pineapple, grapes, or any fruit that had been picked from a bush or tree and not prepared by any manufacturer. That is a foundational truth for stable and long-lasting health.

Gluten free wild oats with juice, seeds, nuts and a little honey. The first thing in the morning was my children's favorite breakfast and is better than any medicine for the immune system.

Prevention on the mental, spiritual, emotional and physical levels is parents' responsibility of course. If we take the extremely important area in our child's life – their teeth, mouth, digestive system, clean liver and kidneys, we will see rapid improvement in their overall health.

Ron Rejects Ritalin

In the early 1990's Ritalin was making big headlines. Even Israeli teachers began to recommend more and more children to use the drug. It is after all a way

Giggling Dr. Green

to help teachers conduct their classes uninterrupted by restless young pupils. However, are drugs ever truly the answer?

Ron seemed to be a very kind and sweet boy. Yet, he had difficulties sitting in class for all the required hours. (I find it very unnatural for young children to sit for so many hours still in class anyways.) Numerous times, his restlessness brought him punishment at school and then further scolding at home. Anet, Ron's mother, was required to meet with the teacher and school administrators to discuss Ron's behavioral problems. Anet was advised the only way he would be allowed to remain in class would be if Ron was administered the new miraculous medication, Ritalin. When Ron received the message, he was very concerned and refused to take any medication. Still traumatized by losing his father to an overdose of a wrongly prescribed medication, Ron was frightened. It had been a terrible mistake, yet all Ron understood was his beloved Father was gone, and medication was to blame.

Anet fully sympathized with Ron 's fears, however she was at a loss for what to do. She tried to reason with her young son, but he refused to listen. The real battle began early the next morning, when Anet tried to give Ron the prescribed dose of Ritalin. With tears in her eyes, Anet pleaded with Ron to take the medication so he could return to his class, however he refused. No punishment was as scary to him as the memory of his Father's last moments alive. Anet missed that day of work and stayed home with Ron. He was perfectly willing to stay home. As the evening approached, Anet felt that something would have to be determined before the next morning. She dreaded another day beginning in battle with Ron, especially since she felt defeated in her empty pleas. Anet sat down with Ron, to explain to him just how important it was that he be able to return to school, instead of the lower grade the school threatened to place him in, and that he must take the Ritalin. Ron spoke with big tears rolling down his cheeks, "Mom, you don't know what this drug can cause. You have not researched or investigated the possible side effects. They scared you at the school meeting, and you did not even question their advice. I need you to know everything about this drug. Not like my dad, who didn't ask, and never investigated. Mom, Daddy is dead. I want you to be able to answer all my questions about this drug, before you give it to me."

Anet felt shame and guilt as she listened to her son, because in her heart, she knew he was right. She stayed home again the next day and, together with Ron, went through all the information she could find regarding Ritalin. The discoveries they made were absolutely shocking to both of them. In her search for an alternative solution, she came to me. My first question was, "Ron, what do you have for breakfast?" Ron told me how much he liked chocolate sandwich cookies along with warm cocoa and marshmallows. And what is your favorite lunch menu? I continued. "Well,", he replied, "I like pizza, soda, and French fries with ketchup. I also like hamburgers and M&M's for dessert. He had a huge smile on his beautiful, intelligent face. He must have known that I would suggest a few dietary changes in order to help him, however, he admitted openly to his vices. We all had a big grin observing his expressions as he gave juicy descriptions of his favorite food choices.

Ron was willing to cooperate with the necessary changes in his diet, and within just one week, his teacher reported significant improvement 'thanks to the miraculous medication'. When Anet returned after one month to meet the teacher, she could see on the teacher's face the expression of, "Didn't I tell you it would make a significant difference?" Of course, Anet kept her and Ron's secret and graciously received the amazingly good reports about Ron.

Ron continues to succeed in school, and faithfully follows his new, healthy way of eating. He was so elated to have escaped taking the dreaded medication that he would have done almost anything. Thankfully, the answer was as close as the fresh produce stand!

Tonsillitis

Karin was hospitalized and one of her tonsils had been removed. She was six years old and had a severe case of tonsillitis during which the doctors told her parents tonsillectomy was their only option. A few weeks later Karin's mother said to me, "had I known better, I would have never let them do that to Karin". Karin was so sure of her parents' good judgment like most young children normally are. The damage to Karin was serious; she lost faith in those whom she had trusted the most. She continued to suffer from different behavioral disorders after that traumatic procedure. The simpler way would be homeopathic methods to help Karin's body to fight her disease and prevent it from recurring. What Karin needed, like possibly all the children in the world, was simply a dairy and gluten free diet. After all, we are not calves, we are human beings. Karin had to attend many therapy sessions to overcome her loss of trust in her personal 'gods', i.e. her parents. The damage of cutting our bodies is irreversible. So, why didn't her parents know any better? Well, Karin's parents, like all parents, worried about their daughter's wellbeing and all they knew was just listening to what the doctors say.

Giggling Dr. Green

This may be a children's question. Yet, all of us parents do the best we can, and the best we know. So, why don't we know more? Why don't we know better? Mainly because we, like our children, trust the 'higher' hierarchy to know better. It is ironic to see the wrongful treatment of a physician's child by other physicians, because even as physicians, some parents simply do not understand the role of prevention.

The most important role is that of prevention. Please do not confuse my definition of prevention with mainstream medicine understanding of prevention. I do not mean any "preventing medications" but responsible and consistent prevention, through healthy nutrition and health promoting lifestyle. This way we can truly remain our child's personal god and be trusted that we do our very best to secure their good health. "Easier said than done", is probably what most parents may say. I do not blame them; in the light of all the commercialized fears and threats, we become paranoid that we do not know anymore what to believe in and whom to trust with our child's health. Well, I was no better or wiser when I was a young mother, and sometimes I had to trust the physicians, also

How tonsillitis can get dangerously complicated

Amanda had recurring bouts with tonsillitis, causing her parents to agree with the doctors, and to subject her to the recommended Tonsillectomy. Although the surgery went seemingly well, the terrifying signs of trouble started only 2 weeks later when Amanda became nearly a vegetable. She suffered terrible headaches that did not respond to any drugs, and in that desperate pain, at only 10 years old, she asked the doctor to let her die.

Her entire nervous system turned chaotic. Amanda could not hold her head up anymore, it just dangled. Nor could she walk, control her hands, or swallow food or drink. Carried in her father's arms she went back to the physician's office. None of the battery tests they ran in the hospital revealed the cause of her desperate and dangerous condition.

When I heard Amanda's story from my friend, a well-known physician, I knew immediately what had happened. Something had gone terribly wrong with the anesthesia during surgery. The administration of the correct choice of homeopathy would have been the only way to prevent the tragic aftermath that anesthesia had produced so I started her treatment with Lach 16 LM

Giggling Dr. Green

And the next remedy was Nux-v 18LM. Those were administered just twice to neutralize the toxic side effects of the medications. Then, I recommended Chiropractic and Cranial-Sacral adjustments.

Amanda's parents, still in awe to realize how terribly their daughter had been damaged by the anesthesia, were ready for homeopathic help. And the relief soon took place.

Her next visit was to a Cranial-sacral practitioner who helped Amanda to realign her upper spine and neck. She recovered from the whole ordeal after only a month. Imagine how much suffering could be avoided had the doctor tried to discover the cause of Amanda's recurring tonsillitis, to begin with. All it would take was a few questions to investigate where her sensitivity came from. After Amanda got better, I had the opportunity to ask her what was troubling her for all those years. The sweet child explained her deep concerns regarding her parents' stressful life, the arguments between them, and the often loud and frightening words they exchanged. She was afraid to lose them. She felt as if she was a heavy financial burden on the family. All of this the young girl told me. Her parents could address the guilt and stress she felt over the family situation. Since she never had the opportunity to say anything, she literally 'choked' and 'blocked' the free blood circulation to her tonsils. How cruel is it to cut the tonsils out, causing horrific suffering, and all in vain, and could be avoided.

Amanda's parents could address the problem in the natural way and avoid the damage she endured, which for too many children is fatal, and would eventually lead her to

How to prevent complications

Mainstream Approach
<u>Antibiotics</u>

Different courses for an extended period of time.

If that does not stop the problem from recurring, move on to invasive measures.

<u>Tonsillectomy (possible side effects)</u>

Emotional trauma

Strep infection

Complications from Anesthesia

Complications from Antibiotics

Giggling Dr. Green

Blood dripping into the lungs can cause death

Accidental death from anesthesia.

Loss of voice

Infectious disease attracted in hospitals

The body will have to find different avenues to signal distress.

The cause has never been removed, only the symptom indicator. The bodies' "Health Alarm" has been disabled. More problems will appear later in life, such as ulcerative colitis, joint inflammations, arthritis, mental disorders, asthma, kidney disease, skin irritations and many other possible symptoms.

My Suggestions

Swollen, red-hot tonsils indicate an acute stage of tonsillitis. The child's temperature will be significantly high, and he or she is unable to eat or drink anything

Please keep in mind that fevers are a natural and even healthy reaction of the immune system in order to restore health. Some children may vomit and cry during the acute stage.

1) Cold washes of the private parts of the child every 1-2 hours, to reduce fever, the redness and the pain.

2) An alternative is a cool wet cloth like a diaper, refreshed every hour.

3) Administer Sulfur 6 LM 10 drops twice a day until the acute stage subsides.

4) If the child is able to swallow, give Lach 6 LM,

10 drops once a day in addition to the Sulfur.

If very restless give Apis 6X (instead) every 2 hours as long as it will serve well. If the child refuses to swallow, giving Graph 8X (instead) would be the choice. If the child is very cuddly and sweet, Puls 6LM (instead) would be the choice.

If the child is very resistant and refuses to be treated, giving Chamomile (instead) would be the choice.

5) In the case of a 'red-hot' face and throat, with violent pain that comes on very suddenly, the remedy of choice would be Belladonna 6 LM, 10 drops once a day.

*** <u>Please do not use the cold washings when administering Belladonna and/or Apis.</u>

6) Please do not give all of the above-mentioned remedies together. It is important to stick to one and let it work for a few hours. The signs of improvement will show up rapidly if you choose the right remedy.

7) If you do not have Homeopathic remedies at your disposal, the cool applications to the private parts will help alleviate the pain, and the body will start the self-healing process immediately.

8) Cool, wet towels, applied on the wrists and ankles will help to lower the temperature in a supportive and gentle way.

9) If the child refuses all food and drink, do not try to 'convince' her or him to eat. The only crucial issue is dehydration. If the child will not drink, the next best way is to drop very small amounts of liquid on the tongue, with a dropper or a teaspoon. The child will then develop a thirst and ask for water.

10) If this does not work for you, prepare a lukewarm bath and let the child relax in the water. The body will absorb the water through the skin, and dehydration will no longer be a danger. During, or shortly after the relaxing bath, most children will start drinking and feel significantly better.

11) ABSOLUTELY NO cold baths to reduce the fever.

12) In case of an extremely high temperature, please add a few grains of sea salt to the drinking water to aid in replenishing the lost electrolytes.

13) Once you are on the right path, it may only take a couple of hours before the child shows improvement and begins to eat and drink.

14) Reflexology treatments are very helpful and efficient.

15) PEMF therapy- is highly recommended

16) Cranial-sacral applications-help the muscles relax and align.

Some children suffer from more serious tonsillitis. I would highly recommend addressing their emotions in those cases. There could be a 'big secret' harboring in their little chest, and they cannot deal with the pain. Not expressing their concerns can create very violent tonsillitis symptoms as well. As far as my experience goes, no antibiotics ever healed sadness, loss or fear. Therefore, help them with Homeopathy, emotional support, games, art and any other way to relax

Giggling Dr. Green

and feel safe enough to reveal their secret. In all cases I would seriously consider a change of diet, especially sugar, meat, dairy and gluten free diet.

A few more suggestions:

1. Gargling with 1 teaspoon Apple Cider Vinegar in a glass of water with a little honey is very comforting. Or the same with just squeezed lemon

2. Plenty of fresh air and sun.

3. Let the child talk and tell you about any fears or anger issues he/she feels.

4. Please do not correct or judge anything the child shares with you, simply listen and be supportive currently.

5. All fruit and vegetables should remain fresh, raw and whole, if swallowing is OK.

6. If swallowing is too painful, simply juice the vegetables, and/or fruit.

7. A cold, creamy fruit puree may be well tolerated, or even frozen fruit juice will help

For the future:

Dairy, meat, gluten free and refined food should be avoided at all times.

Encourage your child to express emotion, either verbally or through art, music or sports.

Provide lots of regular physical activity, especially out in the fresh air.

Drinking plenty of fresh, filtered water every day is vital to good health.

The cold-water washes logic

The thermal auto balance and correction is a very vital asset of every organism. Only even temperature to all parts of the body stimulates blood circulation. In cases of severe hypothermia for example, people may lose their fingers or toes, yet they can still survive because the body's mechanism will supply the inner vital organs with the necessary blood supply and warmth for survival. People can live without a few toes, but the heart and kidneys are vital for existence. The lymphatic fluids move in the body reaching all the inner and outer organs dependent upon muscle and blood vessels peristaltic activity. The accumulated lymphatic fluids cause pain, in this example. In this case I refer to the tonsils (the same is true for any head inflammation) that block the free blood and lymph circulation and inhibit the necessary intensive oxygen supply to the inflamed area. At the same time, this accumulation puts a lot of pressure on the neighboring organs, muscles and nerves. This pressure causes pain as well as slows recovery considerably.

Since we all agree that the body can heal itself, with the cold washes we enhance the blood and so the lymphatic circulation by lowering the temperature at the elimination of organs. In other words, when we create cold shocks to the private organs which are used to expel waste from the body, we create a 'blood rush' to that bottom area, in order to even out temperatures from the cold applications to re-warm it up again. This rush creates a peristaltic motion of the blood vessel; the lymphatic fluid will get into motion that way as well. The abdomen is the place with the biggest concentration of lymphatic nodes. The blood is filtered as it flows through and to the kidneys and intestines and the waste will be driven out of the body, as it should. No, the pressure can be released from the throat and neck area, since the blood and the lymphatic fluid have rushed to the abdomen. That took the pressure off the throat area and opened up the circulation to flow freely again. When the circulation flows freely, the fresh, oxygen-saturated blood can reach the inflamed area. Unhealthy bacteria cannot continue to exist in an oxygen rich environment. This is how the cold washes help the body to heal the tonsillitis and reduce the pain significantly. The same would work for any kind of head and upper body inflammation as mentioned before.

Like sinus infections, headaches, pink eye, eye infections, ear infections etc.

Note: The washes must be short and at room temperature!

Please, keep in mind that these recommendations are very general and may not be the proper remedy for each and every case of tonsillitis. However, the side effects are zero, and it supports the immune system in its natural function. From that point on, the child will be much stronger to overcome the problem. I would highly recommend continuing monitoring the child's improvement, and if it is still not good enough, please call your trusted Homeopath, Naturopath, Chiropractor or Acupuncturist.

In general, for high temperatures, if we do not have the proper Homeopathic treatment to relieve the fever, or we do not want to administer a medication, cool wet strokes over the legs and arms can lower the temperature significantly. The reason is the warm blood cools down as it reaches the capillaries by the cold wet cloth and then returns to the inner body at a lower temperature. This is the best way to support the body in its natural effort to restore health, rather than suppressing the self-healing system with unnecessary drugs and procedures.

Avoiding Surgery

Tali was a beautiful 10-year-old girl. She and her mother just returned from the hospital where they received the very alarming prognosis; Tali would need to undergo hip surgery on both sides for joint relocation. Her mother had heard about me and decided to take a leap of faith and see if anything else other than this invasive surgery was available. I knew with certainty that different avenues existed for Tali. After the first visit the mother said, "Tali is scheduled for surgery in one week".

3 days later, the girl returned, this time with her father, who tried a few challenging questions and asked; "How can you be so sure that Tali won't need surgery, just by your little touches"? I smiled and replied, "At least I won't hurt her, and you can always reschedule the surgery in case we don't succeed. I strongly believe that all Tali needs is just a little support to help release her muscles tension in her hips, so her joints will relocate spontaneously". He asked me how long it might take, and I explained that it should not take more than one or two more applications. The following week, when Tali went back for a checkup with her doctor, to prepare for surgery, the doctor discovered there was no need for surgery anymore. Tali has never experienced a relapse, and resumed a normal active life, as she was a first line dancer in the Israeli folk dancing group.

Tali resumed good health through harmless and non-invasive methods, which enabled her complete health.

The same is true in most cases when children get sick. There are numerous ways to help them naturally, instead of reaching out to the invasive, sometimes fatal and irreversible applications. I know how many parents probably think, "It is very daring and irresponsible of me to voice these opinions". Well, I think it would be irresponsible to keep you in the dark and from this knowledge, brainwashed by mainstream medicine that still uses many of the same philosophies for over 200 years. It is time to reveal the truth of natural, non-invasive options.

Whether mainstream medicine does not know better, or does not care to change, and therefore has no means to treat you or your child differently- is still an open question. This is the reason for their name 'traditional medicine'. Old fashioned, stuck in the dark ages, refusing to open their minds to scientific knowledge proven in the past 50 years by their own peers and medical researchers, and the big money maker notion. The correlations between ongoing scientific research results, knowledge, and ultimately the essential application of this

Giggling Dr. Green

knowledge in the field must be complete for the patient's benefit, rather than the stubborn resistance to these findings, as if they do not exist, and would have no impact on health. Why do the doctors ostracize themselves as if new research does not exist, and uphold the old school ways, so many of which are counterproductive to natural health? Science and medical schools must not stick to the old ways, because it then becomes a history and tradition school, which is appropriate in a church or synagogue, but not in providing for human health services. Let our children be able to trust us, and let us stay open-minded, informed and search for the truth, through ongoing research and increasing knowledge. We must not disappoint our children by holding on to ignorance, blindly following the doctors who received only training to diagnose, and prescribe, but none for supporting the body towards restoring its own health. They cannot even tell what health is. (Read "The cancer answer" by Al Carter).

Severe hip pain at 12

Shay suffered so bad of a shooting pain in his hip that he could not even stand. Well trained as I was in my therapy skills, I was so terribly worried about him (I just had a very disturbing case of a little girl with bone cancer at the same place Shay complained), that I was afraid to assume full responsibility for his care and turned to a Chiropractor. After a few visits, there was no improvement. That did not make it any easier on me, and I lost my confidence to oversee his care even more. Finally, my precious Shay said to me, "Mom, please don't take me to the Chiropractor again. Please, you take over my healing. You know so much more than he does, and I trust only you". I looked at my beloved son, and my heart was torn to the point where I couldn't speak. Yet, I had him lie on the carpet and began to touch his back. Then I pressed a little bit harder, and we both heard the loud crack of relief as clear as thunder. He immediately got up and walked as if nothing had ever bothered his hip, it has never recurred.

Giggling better for Doctors

"If only doctors would keep in touch with their own inner child, they would most likely treat their youngest patients differently."

This is a very sad yet true statement. We were all children born with the gift of a powerful, perfectly planned self-healing mechanism. However, infants receive various vaccinations before they even begin their life path. The alleged reasoning for this assault is; the vaccinations provide better overall health and prevent all the dreadful childhood diseases. Do you believe that? Is your child healthy, or is your child "just one of those" who was harmed by these vaccinations?

According to statistics, there are more children with serious illnesses (like cancer) today than there were 50 to 100 years ago: the same is true for the autoimmune disorders our children are being treated for everywhere in the Western Hemisphere. We hear a lot about the 'Autism Epidemic' in every media, but the true epidemic is not autism, but all the vaccinations and medications forced on our defenseless children. How many autistic children do you know that have never received the mandatory shots? Why do we allow it to continue and let them pretend as if they are searching for answers? Do we really believe in something "out there" causing our children to be so sick and disabled? The amount of funding funneled into those alleged medical research just mocks the underlying truth. Regardless of what the true research results are, the scientists involved will never get th3 opportunity to publicize their findings. They continually hide their results in numerous different politically correct and profitable ways. (Read "Molecules of emotions" by Dr. Pert as she writes about Aids)

It would devastate the autism and vaccination side effects industry beyond recovery. Just consider this. How many people including manufacturers, teachers, therapists, pharmaceutical technicians, care providers, even car plate makers and so on are riding the financial wave of our children's misfortune and misery? This misfortune could so easily be avoided.

Unbearable Suffering

I remember that very desperate mother who called me one day, inconsolably sobbing as she tried to talk to me on the phone. She repeatedly apologized for her endless crying, and we had never even met. Her story is about her 9-year-old son and the unbearable suffering he experienced with daily rivals, anything Hollywood could produce as a horror film. His eyes would never focus, he could not swallow any food, and he was never able to move his bowels naturally. He could not walk, talk, or use his hands. His whole body just rattled and shook constantly, and he was never able to sleep at night. He had an IV connected to him every day. All this went on since he was just one year old, although he had never been involved in an accident and everything in his bright little world had been safe and clean. It was clear to the mother; the vaccinations he had received caused this horrific, irreversible, infinite devastation of his life, if you could even call his painful existence - life. The punch line of her story is as clear

Giggling Dr. Green

an example of bad Karma as I believe I have ever heard; this mother had worked tirelessly for 20 years in the children's department of the Congress fighting for the - Mandatory Vaccination Enforcement bill.

How pathetic - needless to mention, there was nothing I could do to help her.

Greata was 4 years old

was easily the most beautiful child I have ever seen, as if an artist had painted her. She had a very pleasant disposition and easily cooperated as I set about trying to restore her to health, after all the damage vaccinations brought upon her small body. Greta's gorgeous eyes wandered about, unable to focus. Other than to her mother, Greta's limited attempts to speak were indiscernible, her words sounded like a collection of sounds without meaning. Naturally, Greta was embarrassed about not being able to communicate like all her friends. Greta's mother described a normal pregnancy and birth, and that her weight was good. As a baby, Greta was full of life and healthy. However, after the second PDT shot, she started to display some very alarming symptoms - such as severe convulsions and disconnection. The doctors said that everything was OK, and it could be just a "slight reaction to the shot". Yet, after that shot, the "slight reaction" turned into significant brain damage that was irreversible according to the doctor's understanding. By law, Greta had to get the next shot as well, and her condition deteriorated to the point that Greta would never be the normal, bright little girl she was born to be.

It took several months of Homeopathic treatments before we started to see real improvement. Greta received Reflexology treatments as well for an entire year, and the light at the end of her tunnel began to shine brightly. Greta began to say whole sentences, slowly, but clearly. The first time she looked straight into my eyes and said, "I love you", it took every bit of strength I could muster not to dissolve in tears of joy. Her little spirit rose up and joined mine in the battle for her healing. We became very close and working with Greta stopped working, she became part of my heart. I experienced tremendous delight meeting with her twice a week. Greta was so proud when she walked in, in a stable stride, not at all like a toddler anymore. She was able to focus her eyes and hold them straight, and now that we shared eye contact, I could tell she understood how strongly working with her had influenced me personally. Children like Greta, who have very limited verbal communication skills, are able, through the grace of nature, to develop their other senses far beyond the average person. As the year passed, Greta and I formed a team based on trust, faith and desire to succeed only achieved through

Giggling Dr. Green

two hearts bonded for a single purpose. We reached our goals in areas that were miraculous, thank God. I hope Greta will grow up to be a mom herself and will never allow her babies to receive the vaccinations that nearly inhibited her from a fulfilling life.

"Statistics" - Sad excuse

When Judy was an infant, her bill of health was completely normal; however, it took a dramatic downward drop after her second vaccination shot. She began to suffer from very alarming seizure attacks, and her parents had repeatedly rushed her to the emergency room. Her doctor declined any connection between her condition and the shots, since the time between the attacks and the shots was too far apart in his experience. "She should have gotten the attacks right away, usually within 24 hours," said her pediatrician.

Consequently, Judy received her next vaccination as scheduled, and shortly afterwards fell into a deep coma she never recovered from; her brain damage was too radical, yet so preventable.

Judy's parents lost their child to the admitted "statistics" and their grief was over the "only 5%" of children that MEGAForce claims to suffer harm through government-mandated vaccinations. The unfortunate truth, however, is that although your child falls prey to the 5% of ill-affected children you do not care to hear - what a small percentage she or he was - in their statistics, which are terribly inaccurate and are deceptively low, anyways.

Every child is 100 %.

At the age of 8 Joshua was diagnosed with autism because of his restless behavior. He could not attend public school, and his devoted parents had tried every therapy and treatment they could find. Joshua was lucky his parents had the resources to try ways to help him, many parents become trapped in an insurance nightmare fighting desperately for their children 's health needs. Joshua had also great difficulty swallowing even water; when he tried to swallow food it would come right back up.

I began with mercury 6LM for mercury removal and other problems in his blood. It took Joshua's parents by complete surprise to learn that mercury existed in childhood vaccinations. Mercury must be closely examined as a factor in so many brain disorders and damage that vaccinated children have. Mercury contamination seriously harms all cells in our body, including the brain cells causing significantly worse damage as they serve the central nervous system. The restlessness and communication limitations, or, in many cases communication blocks, convulsions, wandering eyes etc. are the result of damaged nerve cells. The central nervous system represents the largest part of the nervous system, including the entire brain and the spinal cord. It plays a fundamental role in control and behavior. Without the nerves, the body will not be able to function at all. We can see it in people who suffer from numbness, or paralysis of any part of their body. The nerves transmit the electric current to activate the muscles; the eyelids for example, open and close only due to the electric current the nerves transmit to the lids. The heart beats only because of the electric current the nerve transmits to its muscle. When the nerves are damaged, or dead, the organs activated by those nerve currents will never be able to function. Bypasses are the body's answer to regenerate the electro-current transmission to the muscle or organ, and very slowly, the person will be able to move and/or activate the organ again.

Mercury is a heavy metal, an irremovable element from the cells. The same mercury exists in amalgam cavity fillings and informed people prefer to have other materials used for their cavities rather than mercury. In the past 20 years, the published information about mercury has motivated a large community of health-conscious people to doubt and investigate many products on the markets for mercury safety.

Joshua's parents finally discovered the best results to his mercury problem were not to be found in the nutrition and chelating therapy, but homeopathy and by electromagnetic field correction of his cells. There are different options for those applications today, and one of them is EMF and vibrational therapy. Walking along the beach every day, or running and playing for a few hours daily, will balance the electromagnetic field of the healthy cells and contribute to cellular metabolism as well. If your child has no access to the beach, do not be discouraged. Hiking in the mountains and woods will help as well. The proximity to nature, without any artificial or manmade materials, and the direct exposure to the open sky, can be of significant help...

Many devices are available to help us improve and recover our healthy cells' electromagnetic field. They vary in price and effectiveness and some of them are highly efficient according to my experience and scientific research. Joshua found undoubtedly significant support and help through the PEMF correction. He went on to graduate high school, served in the army, and went on to college to study therapy for Autism.

He certainly has a good, firsthand understanding of the problem.

Giggling Dr. Green

Born in 1976

A loud and boisterous right from the start. Even the midwife said, "Listen to him announcing his presence. Everyone will know how strong and healthy he is, just listen to his voice already ". He received his childhood vaccinations as required and had no immediate reactions. His mother was so pleased; he never even developed a temperature after the shots. It was not until preschool that the teacher drew his parents' attention to the fact that something was not right with Tal. He could not play at his age level and was not able to sit and listen to a story. He was very restless and always on the go. Even his scribbled drawings lacked age-appropriate details, and his speech was limited to a couple of words. Since he was the youngest in a family of seven children, his parents believed it was just a matter of a spoiled child.

As time went on Tal was due to attend school, and the teacher put even more pressure on the family to have him tested and get a proper understanding of his problem. Test results determined Tal had no pain sensitivity; he would fall and be injured, yet never cry, in fact, after his first vaccination Tal never cried again of pain. He did not develop his fine motor skills at all; he could not build with the Lego blocks and could not manage to hold a pencil or spoon in his hands. He was physically very active, yet only the large muscles. When he reached 12, he could not control his bladder or his bowels yet and developed behavioral problems. While assigned to special education, the school psychologist recommended sending him to a special facility for retarded and emotionally troubled children. His mother refused to send Tal away to that center and chose Homeopathy, Reflexology, natural nutrition and cranial-sacral therapy.

When talking to Tal today, he says, "All I remember from high school is pushing wheelchairs for my classmates. I never learned anything." Tal started reading and writing when he was 21 years old, and by the time he was 27 he was able to obtain and keep a job.

He was determined to be normal, and thanks to his strong will, and the natural treatment he received, he is self-sufficient, living on his own. You would never know today that he was destined to be in the statistics as one of the unfortunate children permanently damaged by mandatory vaccinations. Tal has stated unequivocally that he will never use any medications; homeopathy will always be his only choice when he is sick. Tal continues to work diligently to improve in all areas, and although he realizes his path has been different from his siblings, he feels strong, and up to the tasks ahead of him.

Save the planet for our children
and our children for our planet

Baby's heart failure post vaccination

As I was sitting and writing these lines, my office computer technician approached me. The story he shared with me revealed an even sadder side of the vaccination casualties than I have written yet. He lost his son when he was only 6 months old, due to "an allergic reaction to the PDT shot". The baby suffered major heart damage soon after the second shot and died. This grieving father asked me only one thing, when I requested permission to share his story with you. He said, "Please do everything you can to wake up those parents and caregivers who still believe the vaccinations save our children. They kill the children and debilitate an entire generation".

As he was leaving later, his parting words spoke directly to the heart of my mission. "If only this book existed when my boy was born, I would have never allowed him to receive the deadly shots, and he would be alive today".

These words are so sad, yet so powerful. Today there are growing movements among those who understand the danger of the mandatory vaccination law, and if you take the time to do some research, you will be able to study their findings and receive their updates, enabling you to make a better informed and wise decision for your own children. It would be ideal to gather all this information even before giving birth, so that you have plenty of time to make one of the most important decisions on behalf of your helpless infant. Make the right decision, the intelligent, knowledgeable decision that will protect their health, their life quality and their very future. Please do not procrastinate; do not allow the first shot, and the following shots should not even be considered.

Do not let anyone intimidate you. Your child has the same chance of getting the measles as you do of winning the lotto. However, your child has the same chance to get very ill, become handicapped or die from the shots, as you do-had you cross a busy highway without looking first. That risk is very real, and far too great to take the chance. The exceptions are scarce; children not harmed in any way from the vaccinations are in the minority.

As a parent, you are probably over 20 years old, and you may even be in your 40's. Can you imagine what it would be like to contract chicken pox? How terrible would you feel and how sick would you be? Now, imagine that beside chicken pox, you come down with a whooping cough as well, at the same time. Doesn't it sound like a deadly combination? The high temperature, the severe cough, the terrible sores, the terrible itch so bad that you cannot lie still for a moment. You feel so bad, that all you want is rest and relief that doesn't 'come; you itch, vomit, cough, burn off a high fever, and your chest goes through the worst tearing pain. Now, as if all of that were not enough misery, add to those diseases the pain and suffering an adult experience with the measles. The doctor has just diagnosed you with these three terrible diseases at the same time. You understand as an adult; how serious this news is. With these three diseases together at the same time you are so very ill that the doctor finds it necessary to send you to the hospital, where you just wish you could die. Now, hold on; we are not finished with you yet. Imagine, with the itchy chicken pox, the chest-tearing whooping cough and the miserable, measles-inflicted rash, you don't have enough to struggle with, so we added another disease, polio. Now, you are in the stage of life-threatening diseases. I suppose, with the devastating combination you begin to wish you had never been born, rather than to suffer so terribly. The best-case scenario has you spending weeks in the hospital, and many more weeks at home, recovering from the assault on your entire body. Odds are however, that you will not be so lucky, you have a strong chance of ending up with a handicap such as paralysis from the polio, heart disease from the whooping cough, deafness from the measles, or joint inflammation from the chicken pox. (This is just a fraction of what your child gets when vaccinated with over 39 different diseases.)

Without a doubt, now your immune system is devastated and your struggle just to stay alive would be so overwhelming that your immune system would immediately shut down all other vital functions. The adversely affected hormonal system, along with the unfavorably influenced nervous system, is damaged by all the toxins, disease agents, pain, suffering, high temperature, itching and paralysis.

Would you like to be so sick with all these different diseases at the same time? Would you believe that your whole system would collapse under the painful pressure and breakdown from being so sick? Now, add just 2 more diseases, one is tetanus, and the other hepatitis. I do not think any adult, regardless of how strong or how young, any man or woman would overcome such a health disaster. If an adult contracts any of these diseases, the likelihood of brain damage and or brain function disorders would be very high.

This is exactly what we let the mainstream physicians do to our newborns, as we allow the government to enforce mandatory vaccinations. We don't fight for our children because we are so badly brainwashed; the government has succeeded in convincing us all that it is for - the children's health. What are the chances of any child getting all these diseases at the same time or even in his lifetime? Perhaps one in 20,000,000. What are the chances of any child becoming autistic? A staggering number of six out of 10 and those numbers continue to grow worse each year. According to statistics, boys are more prone to becoming autistic than girls are. Doctors have brainwashed us to believe that if our children did not receive the vaccinations, the exposure to disease would bring certain disasters; however, the real disaster is only in the doctor's office. The MEGA Force cartel is truly not interested in our children's health, whether your child is the victim of their "necessary medications or vaccinations ". Yet, they are fully aware of the alarming numbers and the dangers their drugs place on the victimized children. Their wallets, unfortunately, speak louder than our children's pitiful moans of pain and fear. If you and I believe that they are researching the problem, they will continue to harm, deform and kill millions of our precious kids.

Please consider this; if the vaccinations are so necessary and safe then why are the numbers so alarming? Why do we need ever more and bigger hospitals with more advanced, expensive equipment, and an entire medical industry to care for the increasing numbers of permanently damaged and autistic children? Cancer of those little children, of course, is an even bigger money-making machine. Imagine the economic disaster when the truth about aids, cancer, arthritis, sleeping disorders, autism, multiple sclerosis, etc. is "made known" to the public. Why do I say, "Make known"? Because we each have these truths deep within us, if only we can step away from what we have been taught long enough to remember that we were all endowed as infants with a built-in self-healing mechanism. The only real obstacle for the truth overpowering fear and habit would be by freeing ourselves from the MEGA Force manipulations.

The arguments in favor of mandatory vaccinations continue to be completely ridiculous such as "Well, you don't see epidemics any more like the world saw 100 years ago". Very true; however, bathroom facilities lacked running water 100 years ago, our houses were as good as they were, and please do not forget that our drinking and sewer water pipes have been separated since the discovery of the source of polio-carrying bacteria. When was the last time you saw sewers running along the streets in America? Refrigerators keep the food cool, and doctors have learned to wash their hands or wear gloves between patients. We no longer wash our laundry in the same water contaminated by animal feces, and the water reservoirs are under careful supervision. Our farming fields are no longer fertilized with both manure and human feces, and the marketing of food is also supervised. The whole understanding of personal hygiene has taken a major turn,

Giggling Dr. Green

which contributes to better overall health as well as minimizing the dreaded epidemic outbreaks.

The sad part is children do not get childhood diseases any more, and therefore they have no natural opportunity to develop and build their immune systems. Our children now suffer from what once were considered as - senior citizen diseases. They are developing cancer, tumors, brain disorders, arthritis, ulcers, autism, diabetes, hepatitis and many other horrible diseases. The pharmaceutical companies run their campaigns and advertisements pointing the finger everywhere but - themselves. They cite environmental reasons, viruses, bacteria, pollen, weather, water, sun, soil, pets, food, smoke, etc. I plead with them, please see and admit to the obvious reasons. Humankind is the most adaptable living creature on the planet. People live everywhere on the planet, because we can adjust to any climate, food, manner of pollution, temperature, circumstance, dwelling styles, building material, parental attitude, bosses, families, and tribes. People can adjust to every lifestyle and be very healthy. The sickest people in the world sadly live in America, the most powerful nation that exists today, and the most over-medicated people. Our Congress stands behind the mandatory vaccinations and does not care, as if it were composed of members who are too blind, inhuman and criminal to watch how the nation is getting sicker and sicker by the day, as congress members are too deaf to listen to facts clearly stated directly to them.

I cannot help thinking how shocked the American public was when the truth of the Saddam Hussein regime was published over the media, how ruthless, greedy and cruel he treated his own people. Hello, America, wake up and watch all the suffering right here in our own children's nurseries, unused playrooms and silent swing sets. Our government mandates pain and suffering to our future citizens; by forcing parents to have their babies vaccinated, a process that irreparable damages their immune systems. These poor innocent children, so seriously harmed, are often turning into dysfunctional, handicapped young people and adults. Then, as a follow up to the dangerous, unnecessary vaccination, the government forces parents to submit their child, upon receiving the feared cancer diagnosis, to radiation and chemotherapy. The entire medical community understands these procedures are barbaric and futile. Do they really think we do not know their secret? Another big wake up is needed here, American parents. Everyone thinks cancer is deadly. Not that it really is, but because we were all taught to believe so. Because the medical establishment has worked long and hard to convince us of it, instead of disclosing the truth to us - that this industry is nothing but trillions of dollar revenue generator.

Giggling Dr. Green

Is Cancer diagnosis a death sentence?
(Only if treated by MEGA force)

Sure, **BUT** only because it takes a miracle for the child to survive chemotherapy, radiation, and cruel surgeries. Parents take the responsibility to educate yourselves beyond the mainstream pre-packaged health plans and realize no one knows your children as well as you do. Study your child's best health options independently, including you support your child to heal of cancer - prevent, and treat your child to revive his or her life force and immune system, rather than suppress it even more, as the mainstream does - and kill. I realize that America is so seriously brainwashed, that what I write here seems criminal in many of your eyes. I do understand that so many of you do want the best for your child, yet are concerned about learning and trying anything new, since you "just don't know better". You still want to believe that doctors care more about your children than they do about their bank accounts. Again, I say, "Wake up, American parents", save your children from the worst enemy they may ever face, the MEGA Force. There are members in our government who would probably love to have me strung up, because I am a voice crying in the wilderness, "Wake up, American parents. Open your eyes and realize the danger you are carrying your children into when you take them in your arms to receive their vaccinations". What is the difference between the Saddam Hussein regime where killing the innocent was as common as sand in the desert, and the MEGA Force, killing so many of our children? There is no difference, because you see, the dead are dead, whether one person lines his pockets with the blood money, or many do. If the laws were not such that even parents who want to make the wise choice would not be afraid to have their children removed from their home and they were arrested for child neglect, many more would fight the mandatory vaccinations. Parents stand together and with a collective voice, tell Congress and the greedy doctors and pharmaceutical companies' owners and employees that you demand this medically endorsed massacre stopped immediately. Imagine, with so many sick children, so many dying children, so many obese children, so many diabetic children, so many autistic children, so many ADD children, so many cancers sick children, so many drugs addicted children, what will the great America look like in 20 years? Who will grow up strong and healthy to be the leaders of tomorrow?

What will the biggest concern be in front of Congress in the next few decades? A strong national defense, the US borders, inflation or perhaps global warming? NO, these will all take a back seat to the staggering problem this Nation

Giggling Dr. Green

will face in building and funding enough assisted living facilities for children and youth who have been, and continue daily to be, damaged by unnecessary vaccinations and medications. The strongest and healthiest people in America in the not-too-distant future, will be the older adults, who were fortunate enough not to have received the "magic shots" that became "mandatory "when they were already beyond the age of being ordered to receive them, or the "lawbreaking" children avoiding the shots and medications?

What a sad picture for America's future.

Don't be concerned about what college your child will attend, or what her or his career will be, these hopes and dreams should be secondary to just keeping them healthy enough to go to college or have a career. Don't worry about nuclear bombs or terrorists, they are much more distant threats than your child 's own pediatrician. The FDA exists to protect the nation from dangerous disease transmitters, harmful food additives, and the like. The FDA is there to supervise the food and drug industry, but how pathetic is that? Are they doing a fair and unbiased job, or do the pharmaceutical companies control what the FDA approves of and what will never be available to the desperate public? Why does the FDA disapprove of every natural treatment and application that, "God forbid", could really save children from pain, suffering and death? They condemn and arrest all those who dare to apply any other means than their "authorized" medications, but what is their goal? Could they be helping to establish a sickly nation, absurdly dependent on more and more drugs merely to survive? Why would they endorse building a nation of very sick children who will grow up into very sick adults, if they survive at all? Well, they are on the right path to do just that, victory is on the horizon, because they own the medical industry and benefit from it. However, we do not have to take it anymore: isn't it time to unveil this horrible, deadly, greed driven corruption? Please, wake up, stand with me as I fight to save your children. These medical doctors never learned one iota about health: they only study disease! Of course, for disease, there must be medication, and often surgery, because this is what they learned in the pharmaceutical industry owned medical school. When they look at your child's chart, do they see the joy, the laughter, the tender heart that you see? No, of course not, they see payment on their Hummer, or fully staffed mansion. They see your child with cancer and see a luxurious trip to Europe with their family. Every child is yet another dollar sign to the MEGA Force, nothing more.

Giggling Dr. Green

How long does the good doctor give your poor, sick child? 5 minutes, 10, or perhaps he is a saint and gives 20, which the insurance company recommends. In 20 minutes, does this doctor know more about your child than you do? If you believe that, you have seen too many Hollywood movies, which have taken the greed, corruption and ruthlessness of the medical industry and covered it up with a caring, compassionate mask, one who spends so much time with each patient you begin to wonder if he has more than 2 or 3 patients at all. Forgetting the actors who care about children in the movies, they are no more real than the Tooth Fairy.

Our child is our VIP guest for dinner

I could not possibly tell you how many times I received that question over the years of my children growing up. "How did you make your children love fresh food so much? I can't make my child eat even a cucumber. "We often had family and friends join us for meals, and the answer I was pleased to give every time was simple, "My children really enjoy their meals, and we have a good time while eating."

This must be standard in your home, remember, when children refuse to eat, or have any sort of eating disorder, in most cases unhappiness during meals will be the cause. Remember a Proverb from wise King Solomon, "Better a meal of herbs and vegetables in peace, than a feast in strife". Hunger, appetite, and pure enjoyment of food are very basic natural drives. Never will any species require force-feeding, under normal circumstances. All species on the planet love their natural food when hungry. They will not refuse food unless something is wrong.

When a child is refusing to eat, or must be threatened or bribed into eating, some areas in his life, health or in the home require investigation. For instance, the circumstances, the atmosphere at the table, are conversations pleasant? How are the relations in general around the table? Are there arguments between parents at the table when children are present? If you believe all of these things to be in fine accord, you may look at the environment, and the food itself. Is the child comfortably dressed? I learned of a case where the child had to bathe and dress for bed before dinner. She was embarrassed to eat, sitting at the dinner table in nightclothes. Are the child's clothes appropriate for the home temperature? Is television on during meals? Do you give thanks at the table for the gifts you are about to receive? Are you trying to prepare and serve with love foods from nature's bounty, with plenty of flavor and color? Have you set a pleasant table? Did you encourage the child to help in any way? A child will sit pleasantly with you and help prepare the vegetables, for example, and then be much more willing to try the new ones you serve.

Every meal should be a celebration, a feast of sorts. The content should be very simple, modest, easy to digest, fresh and colorful. Never come to the table angry and rushed for time (most people do). The family around the table is a good cause for celebration. It starts at the first meal a baby receives when he/she "meets" mom. It is the time of which mom should be relaxed, if possible, to make the baby feel confident and secure. I know we do not live in a bubble. Yet, regardless of how much stress we face, or even how many people are around the table, there is no excuse for hurried and unpleasant meals. The first meal and every meal after should be served in the softest, safest cocoon we can possibly offer. Make your table a safe nest for your family, no matter what they face during the day, let them know when they are around your table, happiness, gratitude and that they are loved. Look at the animal kingdom and notice how the female will not allow any stranger near her and her young ones at mealtime. We are responsible for our baby's eating habits and their digestion. Creating healthy eating habits starts right there when the baby is just born. Which creature in nature will eat when the noise is so bad that they cannot hear their own breath? In nature if you cannot hear your own breath that means that you cannot be relaxed and content and certainly cannot hear a predator nearing you. To be relaxed and content you had better have a quiet and peaceful environment. How many times do we hear "I can't eat? I am too nervous or upset "?

When a child is sad, he/she cannot eat or is very nervous, stressed and frustrated; the children will still sit in front of the TV and gobble down anything in their reach. We need to teach these young people respect for their body. We need to encourage them to bless the food and be very grateful for having food. Food is not a solution for any negative emotions or attitudes. To be sure, we can define the difference; we must learn it ourselves and then teach awareness. The time it takes to prepare a nice meal, and set a respectable table is what Mother Nature deserves for providing our family with the food we have been given. This should be a time of reflection and preparation, and a time to fill our hearts with joy and love. We can teach our children from early on how relaxing and enjoying our food is and more important than anything else while at the table. It is the time of reaping the fruit nature provided for us, which gives us sustenance for life. I cannot stress enough the importance of this process that seems so easily taken for granted. Eating in front of the television, or just mindlessly swallowing something quickly while playing a video game will not generate healthy digestion, appreciation for the food, or the family bonding that only happens during a meal.

Giggling Dr. Green

I have learned from an old friend that the best way to learn to relax and help our body to utilize the nutrition to the best is to take a single, perfect grape and look at it. Enjoy the color, and drink in the marvelous scent. Now put the grape into your mouth and hold it there for a few moments. During this time, do not become occupied by anything else, simply experience the grape in your mouth, and begin to visualize the seed it grew from, the soil that enveloped it for the whole season. Consider the time it took to grow and imagine how the rain and sun helped the wine grow. The fresh air and sunshine brought about the sweetness of that grape. Do not forget the vineyard, so vast, with so many clusters of grapes, but out of that whole vineyard, you have this one, lovely grape. Try to think of as many descriptions as you can for this perfect little grape. Sweet, juicy, round, smooth, with a soft inner part…! Feel it with your tongue; now begin to take just tiny little nibbles of it, and let it go down your throat slowly, experiencing and appreciating all the blessings this grape is bringing to your very fiber. It is going to nurture your cells, your body and if you have allowed it to, your heart and soul, as well.

It is unrealistic to spend all this time and thoughts on one grape regularly, certainly, but if you remind yourself of all that is to be appreciated about a single grape, it will improve your entire attitude about food, consequently blessing your whole family with calmness, peace, and joy you serve with each meal. No child would have any eating disorders if we parents devote more calm and positive energy at the times we serve their food. Young children are happy to help with the meal preparations yet; we do not always have the patience or tolerance to allow them to do so. Softly and quietly speaking during the meal preparation brings that same tone to the table. I promise you that no one in your family will

overeat, or refuse to eat, in such a setting. Shay, Maayan and Tal even picked the fruits and vegetables from our fields, to bring them home, and never had any eating problems.

Remember how good the food tasted when as a child, your family went on a picnic? What is the great magic in picnics? Why does the food taste so much better; why do children love them so much? The fresh air, the fun, family day - even just a bread crust - would taste like heaven. Examples such as picnics are the best proof of the good atmosphere needed for children to thrive. They are so happy, vibrant, enthusiastic, helping, taking part in the preparations, carrying heavy stuff they would complain about at home, and pleasantly cleaning up after the meal. Children are very sensitive to their environments. Please remember, your children do not care if the furniture is of the highest quality or that your table linens are expensive. No need to mention the price of food to them; the sensitive child will stop eating to save you money. All they need is a big smile when coming to the table, and a meal served with love.

Even just rice with beans will be gobbled down as a feast meal

Keep the dinner peaceful and smiling

Everyone in Sarah's family suffered from digestive disorders. When I sat down to go over her eating habits and mostly served meals, she shared with me the tension, anger, sadness and misery at the family table when she was a child. "Every time we sat down together, my father just seemed very angry. He never stopped yelling at us to mind our manners and we were scared of him. He would suddenly hit the table with both of his big fists, and we would all shake in fear. Then he would look around the table, and choose one of us, sending him to eat alone in the bathroom, as punishment for imperfect behavior. He could scare us even just by looking at us as we could never, please him. If one of us held the fork incorrectly, or his mouth closed properly as we chewed the worse anger burst would fall on us. Dinner was also the time he would scold us for anything else going badly in our lives, schoolwork especially. Getting together around the dinner table was a nightly ritual in terror for all of us, and the food would just stick in our throats; when we were able to swallow, our stomachs would crunch and hurt and be upset all night."

With such a sad story, no wonder why these children grew up with ulcers, colitis, asthma, irritable bowels, constipation, concentration difficulties, intolerance and sensitivity to other people's eating habits. As adults they continued "the tradition" of terror with their own families, following the destructive example they experienced. Only with deep personal cleansing, and forgiveness to their father, could those damaged children finally grow up and conduct peaceful meals with their own families. They understand now how vital it is; to avoid disagreements at the dinner table, kindly guide their children towards better manners, have a good sense of humor, maybe soft background music and an attitude of gratitude for the food.

German manners and small pleasure

My parents left Germany right at the beginning of WWII. My father was a very German style meticulous table manners man and was proud of the way we handled the knife and fork at dinner correctly at the age of 4. I knew how important it was to him, and I am grateful for the way he helped us, wisely with

Giggling Dr. Green

his great sense of humor to learn proper eating manners. He never scared or
intimidated us, and certainly never yelled at us at the table. Instead, he found a
funny way to make us "follow the German rules at the table". (Only when I was
60 years old, did I learn that my father was not even German at all; he was
Czechoslovakian!)

Growing up in Israel after the Second World War was a very harsh lesson
for a happy little eater such as I was. I have been very slim my entire life so it may
be hard to believe how much I love to eat. Israel was in a deep recession then.
Clothes and medical supplies were in short supply, there were very few cars seen
on the streets, but above all I remember the lack of food. The market shelves were
bare, food rationing was in effect and some foods were very scarce and required
special health needs to be eligible to obtain at all. For my 4th birthday, I received
the best gift from my father, a whole apple, just for me. I will never forget the
smell of that beautiful, red apple. My aunt, whom I dearly loved, would bring us
her monthly banana rations. They were so hard to get, one of those foods for
people with special needs my uncle qualified for. For years I could not explain my
obsession with ripe bananas. I have never had a problem with any food; I could
take or leave desserts, cakes, candy etc. However, oh, if I spy a ripe banana, I will
lose all my manners, come right out, and ask for it! Bananas will always remind
me of family, comfort, joy, a treasure to be cherished and enjoyed at every
opportunity. They must have the beginning of the dark spots to complete my sweet
memories.

The reason for this long-drawn-out discussion on bananas is to show the
association with food and its significant role in our development. Therefore, if we
want our children to love a certain food, we better tie it to the best emotional
association as we possibly can. This is the case with every food we serve on the
table.

When our children were very young, and a certain fruit or vegetable
would be essential for their health in my opinion, I would take it and put it just on
my plate. That immediately would raise their little voices: "And what is for me?"
Instead of saying: "It is very important and healthy for you". I would say: "Sorry,
this is just for me". This way the children became eager to get the same.

The most expensive food, served in the most elegant dining room, will
never have a healthy impact on our children if the atmosphere at the table is

stressful and harsh. Also, when a well-intentioned grandmother serves fruit, after a heavy meal to her grandchildren should not wonder why these children hate fruit?

Omrie has been a great eater since she was very young. Though she has a very skinny feature, one would not suspect her good appetite and love for fresh fruit and vegetables, food she can never have enough of. When Omrie was with me, she could gobble down an entire berry basket declining any sharing, which in any other way is very unlikely of her character.

Vegan

When Omrie was little her mother always let her help with dinner preparations, and the table was nicely set for both. Omrie was a slow eater, and her mother would finish her plate way before Omrie. At that point Omrie had to watch her plate, because mom would "help" her finish faster by picking from Omrie's plate. Omric learned to eat faster since or else she would have to give up on her meal for her mom. It was very funny to hear this little 2-year-old saying: "Mom, you steal my food." Mom would reply with a big smile and was forgiven. But, boy, did that teach Omrie to cherish her food.

It is completely unnecessary to serve expensive food to your family. Price is no indication of nutrition value, the opposite is true, the simpler the healthier and richer in nutritional properties. Your child is not impressed by serving high ticket gourmet meals but prefers the colorful juicy natural raw food. Children are God's greatest expression of the beauty of nature. Why, then, is the food America serves at a typical meal so unnatural? As beautiful little natural people, children would easily grow to love natural foods. If we begin to teach our children to respect their bodies, and feed them accordingly, their future health concerns will be rare. If children start their "gourmet" adventures with the earth's most simple and basic foods, they will develop an absolute love for the best foods available. People are advised to return to these natural foods when they are diagnosed with horrible diseases. So why not practice preventive medicine?

Well, if you are waiting for a representative from the MEGA Force to help you learn about good, safe, natural nutrition for your family, I hope you have the patience of Job, because it may never happen. Most doctors in America are not going to explain the simple truths about feeding your children healthy, natural and above all safe foods but I will; I have no monetary investment in the chemicals and growth hormones injected into our food to produce quicker weight gain in the cattle, chicken, fish, etc. If the saying "You are what you eat"- is true, and I believe it is, then do you really want to feed your child artificial chemicals and growth hormones, causing countless health problems including premature aging cancer and obesity? Most doctors in America have no clue what good nutrition is; they did not study it and all they really learn is what prescription to write for ulcers, indigestion, diabetes, arthritis, liver cirrhosis, kidney malfunctions, and so on. How about preventing all those disorders? I understand that doctors never study healthy nutrition; they were probably not raised on healthy nutrition, the correlation between natural food and long-lasting good health - does not exist. If you took the time to read through the current medical school curriculum, you would find nothing among the diverse descriptions describing proper natural nutrition as a reason for all the modern culture diseases, and possible means to avoid all that illness.

In the nutrition books published by the Food and Drug Administration, dairy and meat products, for example, are highly recommended. That certainly falls in line with what most of us grew up being told by our parents, doesn't it? Dairy products are necessary for healthy bones and teeth; milk does the body good, right? No one mentions how devastating these dairy products really are for our child's health and our own health. The myths that dairy products are "good for your bones" are pathetic. If that is true then why, in America, where dairy products are abundant and affordable for everyone, do we struggle so desperately with osteoporosis, osteoarthritis and bone fusion problems, kidney stones, kidney malfunction, kidney shut down, heart disease and the list go on forever? These are huge money-making industries, with surgeries, prescriptions and over the counter drugs ordered constantly by doctors to correct, or at least alleviate, a generation of milk drinkers and dairy consumers, of their pain. Why don't we stop a moment and consider what part of the picture does not make sense, even to us 'less educated people '?

Israeli newspapers have published numerous articles about girl's premature hormonal development, as young as 8 and 9 years old. These young girls are developing breasts, and begin their periods so young because of the growth hormones and medications the cows had been fed. People are developing cancer in alarming numbers, and the poor children are diagnosed with breast and prostate cancer at the ages of 8 to 11 years old. These articles went on to explain how many children were born with malformed sexual organs, again, attributed to being the results of medicated dairy product consumption.

Do you still believe your children need dairy products in their diet? A completely dairy and meat-free diet has been proven to be the only healthy nutrition and supplies all the needed calcium, minerals, proteins, carbohydrates and vitamins, without any need for supplements. This natural eating should not even be called a diet, which has a negative connotation for many of us, so let's call it - simply a healthy lifestyle. In a later chapter, I will recommend a few recipes rich in calcium for normal healthy bone growth that will not put your child in any medical harm. The hormones and antibiotics that bring about fast growth in cattle and the fight of their infectious diseases save money and grow profits, but at our children's expense. They have also been given to the dairy cows to produce an unnatural amount of milk. These same hormones penetrate our bodies and create almost the same reactions. However, we are not cattle; we do not need to gain weight in a short time or produce more milk and neither do our children. The government's efforts to find the cure for the nation's number one epidemic, obesity; how ironic is that? This same government has not prevented the pharmaceutical companies from production of these hormones for the dairy cows and cattle. Are we so naïve to believe that they do not know exactly what the real reason for the obesity epidemic is?

Though we cannot fight the establishments face on, since there is too much big money involved and the Dairy, Meat and Drug industries will never change unless it is for bigger profits, never to merely enable healthier children. We do have the power to control our own children's nutrition in order to lead them to absolute good health into their future. We have to make these changes in our own homes, at our own tables. We must raise our children safely in this world of "money versus health". We are obliged to protect our children by feeding them the best food possible, not the commercialized over-processed, less nutritious foods yet over medicated and pesticides, we are brainwashed to serve. This MUST stop.

Good food is the food that creates life. For the past 60 years, I have been preaching to anyone who was willing to listen that "live food gives life". In my younger years I made many mistakes, (of course, who hasn't?) and expressed my thoughts even to those who were not asking for my opinion. One of these was my mother-in-law. She was a typical good mom, who would put all her time and energy into cooking fine meals for her family. Everyone in her family praised her cooking, and it was an established tradition that Friday night dinner was at her house. She was a heavy woman herself and was so proud and happy to see how pleased and satisfied the whole family was with her delicious dishes. Everyone but me; I could not eat anything she served, which naturally made me an outcast in the family. However, what could I do, I could not even stand the smell of her cooking, let alone eat it and risk becoming very sick. It was no surprise to me how, she as well as her children and grandchildren were all sick with ulcers, fungus, cancer, asthma, hemorrhoids, gallbladder stones, prostate problems, constipation, varicose veins, bladder problems, sleep apnea, etc. One day I had the nerve (and poor tact) to say to her, "It is so interesting how much time and effort women spend in the kitchen to make their whole family sick". That was so bold and ill-mannered of me to say. Especially to a kindly, simple woman who strongly believed that she was doing her best for her family. I now realize that although I still believe in the basis for my statement, it was a dreadful way to go about saying it. Still, her same mistakes are being duplicated by her off springs and in countless homes across America every night, as moms spend so much time, energy and effort to cook and serve their family meals that will only ruin their health. Oh dear, perhaps at this point a few of you are considering tossing this book into the fireplace or the nearest dumpster!

Well then, for those of you who continue to read, and I thank you for your tolerance, I do suggest you plan your dinner. However, if you really want to have a healthy, happy family, please learn how to stay as close to the original nature of the produce as possible and remember, "Live gives life" which has been my motto my entire life. "A natural plant-based food a day keeps the doctor away".

For many years, I had no solid, written proof to guide my listeners for them to believe me and accept my concept. Until I happened to read the book "The Field: The Quest for the Secret Force of the Universe in 2003, by famed author and journalist, Lynne McTaggart. In addition to her marvelous books, McTaggart and her husband Bryan Hubbard are directors of a public company called "What Doctors Don't Tell You Ltd," which publishes insightful newsletters and books in the alternative health field.

In her book, she documents research done about the true light we all have in our body. Would you believe that scientific research has found a way to measure the light in our cells? The most beautiful and exciting part of this research for me was the explanation of how light gets into our cells, and what the benefits of it are for our health. Believe me, I realize this may sound a bit bizarre to you but is now proven as solid of a fact as gravity. This light in our cells comes from the fresh plants we eat. The water from the plants flushes out of the body and the light stays in our cells. I do not believe this to be the appropriate place to elaborate much further, but I highly recommend reading the book. It is fascinating to find the truths we would never hear in any doctor's office, or in any hospital. Now then, won't you please give a second thought before preparing your beloved child's dinner?

Would you believe me if I said that, there could not be any light in a slaughtered cow, chicken, pig, lamb, or fish? I do not believe that any dead food can give life. The same is true about processed and "factory foods".

Giggling Dr. Green

If we say, "we eat meat" it sounds as referring to a meal, however, try to say: "I prepared dead animals for your dinner, honey".

Would you be surprised if I now mention the same lack of life energy or life force in all the commercialized and over-processed food? This is one of the worst crimes that big business has ever committed against the public. Their recklessness required them to work in the factories, where secret formulas are disguised as food and sold for the purpose of feeding our families and pets. May God forgive them; they know not what they do.

Fresh vs. Formulated or processed

Real food is - what we would have eaten 400 years ago. "Macaroni cheese " did not exist 400 years ago, but brown rice did. Orange juice did not come in a carton, you had to peel and eat the fruit from the tree. Spinach was available 400 years ago, but it was not cooked beyond all taste and nutrition and canned in salted water. Soda did not exist, and neither did energy drinks. A good day's work, a freshly prepared meal, plenty of cool water, and an evening walk replaced the need for caffeine, sugar and then sleeping pills to help us fall asleep.

Corn syrup is an industrial trick used to hook our families on many kinds of processed food. If you suspected that corn syrup is addictive, you were completely correct. The business of new food engineering is deeply entrenched in the ability to hook people on certain foods for their profit margins, not for our children's health.

If we now understand that processed food is not fit for human consumption, or perhaps we should try to understand what these UFOs (unidentified food objects) are good for. They serve one purpose and one alone. UFOs bring health to nothing other than the bank accounts of the manufacturers, the designers, the advertisers, the packaging plants, and eventually, the medical industry. These nutrition deficient "foods" keep our children sick, as they grow up to be sick adults, which is a win-win situation for all the afore-mentioned individuals, and at the end of it all, the MEGA Force steps in to offer a pill, surgery or both, to correct the years of unhealthy eating. If we look into a bleached rice bag, or into the quick oats or spaghetti package, you can rest assured that insects will never grow. Insects are sensitive to chemicals.

Giggling Dr. Green

The best foods to serve your family are not difficult to find, nor are they expensive, and blessedly, require little or no special preparations. Have you ever taken your children to an orchard, or to a vineyard, and let them run free and happy in the fresh air, drinking in all the beauty, and drenching their beautiful little faces in fresh fruit as the juices flood their faces with pure natural goodness? During one of my recent visits to a health food store in Florida, it occurred to me how differently children grow up in the city than they do in more agricultural areas. I observed a little boy who was sitting nicely in the shopping cart anxiously waiting for his chosen treat. His mom checked out and handed her child a green cylinder-shaped container, full of what seems to have been a potato at some point in time. The boy was so happy and excited when he opened the container and started his feast. At that moment I dropped the coin. As I walked to the car, I recalled the joy of my son, Shay, every time we took him to the orchard. I carried little Shay on my back, and he was so happy. He made very loud lip-smacking noises, such as you would hear when a child bites into a perfectly ripe, juicy orange. He would not stop until I lifted him up high enough so he could pick his own orange. Did I mention my back was drenched in orange juice? It sure is a small price to pay for such a wonderful memory. Our boys grew up very fortunate to run after dad in our fields, picking their own tomatoes, bell peppers and oranges. They even knew how to break a watermelon open in the field and just dive into the juicy sweetness. I am so glad our boys did not grow up thinking that oranges grow in cartons, or that parsley is just for decoration on a restaurant plate, or that tomatoes grow on the supermarket displays and eggs just come from the refrigerator. They grew up without having to celebrate the artificially green colored and processed snack container. Their little legs did not dangle down in the supermarket cart. They ran through fields, orchards and all manners of nature. I realize that this is not every child's reality. Not all children grow up in a village to the south of the Dead Sea, but every child should learn to enjoy nature's gifts, to the best of our ability and not just learn from early on that; "Cows give us meat and milk, chicken give us eggs and meat, to grow to be healthy big daddy's." Stop buying into these misleading health destroying lies.

When labels read: - "no additives and no MSG. All natural flavors", we better teach our children that this is not nature by any means. For our sake, keep in mind that we are natural beings, and as such, the only way to stay healthy is by eating natural food. Healthy food simply grows; it does not require a degree in food engineering to produce it. I recall hiking with a friend of mine in the Rocky Mountains and was very excited when I found wild strawberries. As I was reaching to pick one, my friend screamed out loud: "Don't eat that, you don't know if they are safe!" I got a good chuckle from looking at his panicked face, but then as I ate a few, exclaiming on the wonderful flavor, he asked, "Do you really think they are alright, should I try them?" I answered with a humorous tone, "Well, why don't you wait a few hours and see if I am still alive first?" All kidding, aside, however, if you are not familiar with the different plants you may discover in your area, do make an effort to learn about them before trying any, and especially before offering any to your family. There are many good books available on gathering wild foods, including flowers, and so-called weeds, so invest in one and carry it with you until you feel you have a good knowledge built up.

You will never regret allowing your children to learn where true food comes from, so take short drives, if necessary, visit organic farms and let your children enjoy the chickens, the colorful fruits and vegetables, and the fresh air. I would be happy to know that all children are educated about the truths of dairy and meat and help them to make healthier choices for themselves.

Chapter two

Good food can definitely heal, as much as processed food can harm.

Many well-written books available cover this subject extensively; however, I do want to get you started with some of my personal favorites.

All fresh fruits and vegetables are rich in vitamins, minerals, proteins, healthy sugar, essential oils, antioxidants, fiber and healing properties.

Fruit

Apples

Do you recall the saying, "An apple a day keeps the doctor away"?

Well, it is very true. The apple's richness in pectin, fiber, vitamins, iodine and kaolin makes it a very important ingredient in our child's healthy nutrition.

Fiber and kaolin are vital for the digestive system health.

Seeds are rich in iodine and have traces of cyanide for our immune system.

Vitamin C

Giggling Dr. Green

It is rich in Pectin- to support a healthy immune system. For a wonderful start to the day!

Apricots

Very rich in vitamins, especially in vitamin A and C. Absolutely delicious and beneficial for a stable and well-functioning immune system.

Dried apricots are very nutritious yet, it is important to buy the uncultured, unsulfured variety only. Or dry the fruit yourself.

The dried apricots are a good choice for a snack instead of any fast-food snacks or different kinds of chips. (Please be careful with Diabetes for the relatively high sugar).

Apricots alleviate many different types of lung complaints and conditions such as asthma, useful for treating anemia due to their high copper and cobalt content.

Avocado

Rich in vitamins, and enhances the production of vitamins A and D.

A source of good healthy fat and a terrific ingredient for making natural ice cream.

Good for the skin by consumption or, even as external application.

Helps to clean the saturated fats in the blood vessels

Rich in Omega 3. Good for intestinal functions as well as for the nervous system and brain functions.

Supplies a good balanced combination of moisture and fats and so easily absorbed.

Binds easily with oxygen and helps the body to maintain rich oxygen cells.

Avocado is easy to prepare and tastes delicious, sweet, sour, or spicy

Banana

Bananas are rich in potassium, (which helps with hypertension) and helps to regain energy and inner warmth. They are a complete source of nutrition, regardless of how much you eat.

Bananas replenish vitamins, like E, B6 and B12.

Very helpful for histamines balance and can help to ease diarrhea.

Giggling Dr. Green

Bananas help to calm down coughs that do not seem to stop. Ripe bananas are useful as a complete, healthy food as well as a good pharmacy. Helps to lubricate the intestines, detoxify the body, and manage sugar cravings.

Berries

All berries are very nutritious. Even bears love them and thrive on them. Berries are very high in vitamins and antioxidants and, if fresh, are true treasures on every plate.

They are one of the most recommended fruits for better health and a highly active immune system, even if they are at times a little tart.

Cherries

Cherries are good for arthritis and rheumatism; they are rich in iron, which improves blood oxygenation. They create nice body warmth, which may be the reason for their popularity in cold countries. They are very rich in vitamins.

Cranberries

Cranberries are the most efficient kidney cleansing remedy, rich in vitamins and pectin. Cranberries are an important part of every health-oriented nutrition plan. They are very useful for bladdeinfekidney disorders, and many skin and lung disorders. I would not recommend using the canned fruit or bottled juice unless it is definitely fresh-squeezed with no sugar and additives. Good for all ages. I like to cook them very briefly, just until they pop, with only fresh orange juice and maple syrup makes a great jelly.

Dates

Dates are complete nutrition with all we need for daily healthy nutrition.

They are cultivated in desert areas, all over the world. The dates serve the desert people sometimes for weeks and even months, replacing any food. People can live off dates and water, and will still be nourished.

Best healthy snack you can get. I use it to prepare flour, sugar and oil free cookies.

Enhance the immune system and taste delicious, while very rich in antioxidant

Figs

Like dates, figs are the most perfect and complete nutrition. Along the Mediterranean countries figs, dates and water are considered as wholesome nutrition. Figs are rich in iron and vitamins, and aid in all types of digestion disorders. I would highly recommend not over indulging in figs, but a few a day can contribute to your child's health dramatically.

Start your child off with healthy snack habits, and figs would certainly be included in that effort.

Grapes

Grapes serve as significant health enhancing nourishment.

In the past few years, unfortunately, the genetic engineering industry found it very attractive to grow seedless grapes. The best grapes are those with the seeds. The grape seeds play an important part in our PH balance as well as in the antioxidants supply. If you could juice a few grapes a day with the seeds intact for your child, and have him/her drink it, for their immune system - it would be very valuable.

When antibiotics and all the steroids do not help, fresh grape juice, or even just fresh grapes, can help in cases of recurrent inflammations. Grapes are cleansing and beneficial for regenerating the body's ability to create all the vitamin B complex. Traditional Natural Medicine has long suggested fasting on grape juice and fresh grapes for 10 days and even more, and there have been countless reports of individuals with diabetes healing during grapes fast, as well as all infectious diseases.

Grapefruit

Although sometimes slightly sour and can even have a little bitter taste, it is still the best citrus fruit available. Unlike the orange that is much sweeter, the grapefruit is alkaline producing. As such it is an important fruit for better digestion and elimination, as well as rich in vitamin C, for the immune system. The grapefruit is ancient and is an important treasure for everyday and everyone's use and enjoyment. (Sadly that this needs to be mentioned in a children's natural health promoting book, but the reality is that many children these days take medications that create damaging reactions when grapefruits are consumed. So, please pay attention in case your child is on such medications).

I would never recommend bottled or canned grapefruit, but fresh only.

Grapefruit will help with poor digestion, increases appetite during pregnancy, helps to alleviate intestinal gas, and reduces mucus conditions of the lungs.

Lemon

Giggling Dr. Green

Lemon - resembles the grapefruit in its alkaline producing properties, and not acidic like the orange- in spite of its tartness. Lemon serves for a superb dressing for every salad and for healing and prevention purposes as well. It is an absolute must have in every home as a medicine for many illnesses. Do not use bottled lemon juice; it's harmful and useless. Lemon peel, chopped very fine, will enhance every salad, and every cake or cookie. The lemon is simply invaluable. Best medicine for a cold, sore throat, overeating, hoarseness, stings, etc.

Olives

Another fruit cultivated in the Middle East and is very healthy and important in our nutrition. Olives are rich in unsaturated oil, and the cold pressed unfiltered olive oil is the best oil for a healthy nutrition. Olives are best when they are ripe and pickled. The little bitter taste indicates the healing essential oils for the digestive system benefits. The extra virgin cold pressed olive oil serves in many traditional countries surrounding the Mediterranean Sea for numerous healing purposes. For example – gallbladder stones removal, artery cleanser, skin, health services etc. Every health oriented household should keep good olives and olive oil. Olive oil will not saturate in cooking and frying. Although it is a little more expensive than the vegetable oils, it is well worth the difference. Olives are very healthy for their Omega 3 as well as probiotics for the positive microflora in the intestines. Olives help with digestion and are rich in protein and good fat. The best tasting olives come from the Middle Eastern countries, in a huge variety of colors and tastes.

Olives are a whole food and you could survive with water, olives in case you had.

Papaya

Balances the inner secretions of the stomach and acts as digestive aid. Papaya also helps to moisten the lungs and alleviate coughing. It contains carpaine, a phytochemical that cancer cells despise. Papaya is very rich in vitamins and all other needed nutrition properties to promote good health.

Pear

A healthy fruit rich in vitamins and its seeds contain absorbable iodine through the digestive system. Easy to digest and enhances the immune system. A great snack sweet and an absolute health treasure.

Pineapple

Pineapple is rich in vitamin C and very healthy and delicious when used fresh vs. canned.

Giggling Dr. Green

Pineapples are a whole food, since they contain everything the body needs.

Prunes

Low in calories, and makes a good sweet and healthy snack, while aiding digestion.

Helps to prevent constipation more effectively than any medication with no harmful side effects.

When fresh fruit is not available, prunes serve just as well.

Rich in potassium and fiber.

Raspberries

Raspberries benefit the liver and kidneys, help clean the blood of toxins, and are useful in treatment of anemia. They are rich in vitamins and antioxidants. It would take many pages to mention all the berries' health benefits.

Watermelon

The refreshing effect of fresh watermelon on a hot summer day is one of the biggest gifts nature has bestowed on us.

Yet, there is more to the watermelon than just that delicious refreshment we all love. Watermelon is the healthiest and most harmless kidney cleanser ever. If your child suffers from any kidney malfunction, such as slow and insufficient urination, bladder infections, dehydration, fluid accumulation, etc. Watermelons can do wonders. You do not need to serve a lot of it. At times just a little bit of watermelon juice, fresh of course, will do the trick. The urine will start to flow freely and in high volume. When we urinate sufficiently, the burning pain in the urethra quickly subsides. Some girls, at a very early age, develop vaginal fungus. Watermelon relieves the suffering of vaginal fungus in a safer and more effective way than any vaginal creams and antifungal pills, etc.

For children who suffer from high fever and refuse any food or fluids, cold watermelon would be an important fruit to have on hand, because it will supply a little fructose, some electrolytes and the cool fluids the child needs. It tastes a million times better than any medicine.

The list of healthy fruits is endless and each fruit helps and contributes to perfect health.

Giggling Dr. Green

Please see every fruit as a healthy food, healthy snack, and a gift from nature.

Please start your child's day with a ripe fruit, instead of manufactured cereal and milk. These are the most harmful breakfasts I can think of, besides the pancakes, eggs and ham, or a glass of milk. A fresh fruit juice with sugar free and vitamin enriched free cereal can replace any other day start, for best health, for good concentration and performance.

Vegetables

This is a short list for a well of endless health resource
Asparagus

Good for kidneys, and fight fungus.

Very helpful for uncovering hidden emotional issues and makes it so much simpler to heal.

Healthy low calorie snack.

Served raw, asparagus is very good for your digestive and urinary systems.

Beets

Beets are traditionally recognized as "Cancer cells number one enemy". Ancient medical literature emphasized the importance of fresh beets in everyone's diet, and even more importantly in cancer treatment diets. Beets are very rich in vitamins and minerals and the antioxidants in them are of huge importance. In my own natural health practice, I have witnessed people succeeding to eliminate and dissolve tumors by juice fasting with beets, carrots, celery, and kale. I highly recommend adopting different beet dishes from various cultures, to enhance the body's abilities to fight any disease.

Bell pepper

Though very healthy, they need to be ripe when picked and should not be consumed when genetically engineered. Like the tomatoes, they are rich in vitamins and fiber, yet only under natural growing conditions. Like the tomato, you can grow them in flowerpots in every sunny and ventilated space.

The Bell pepper is a very healthy, somewhat sweet crunchy snack children would gladly munch on, because of its delicious taste and has healing qualities.

Cabbage

Giggling Dr. Green

When I studied for my Natural Health exams, I read a book that was entirely about cabbage. There is not enough room in this book to tell all the miraculous healing assets this wonderful food boasts.

However, I will whet your appetite for this bundle of health with a few tips:

Fermented cabbage, commonly called sauerkraut, replenishes the positive microflora in the intestines that helps to recover the B12 production in the body for the recovery of the immune system. B-12 takes part of the hemoglobin creation, our oxygen container and transporter in our blood.

Cabbage leaves put on a sour stomach, boil, aching head, inflamed knee, etc, will relieve the pain. When the pain is relieved, the blood circulation flows freely again. That free flow helps the lymphatic fluid transfer the acidity to the intestines and the bladder, which helps the knee heal. This is because when the knee does not hurt any more, it means the swelling went down, and when the swelling goes down it indicates that the lymphatic fluid is flowing and is no longer accumulating in the knee tissue. That enables the blood to remove the toxins and the acids and supply fresh blood rich in oxygen to the sore knee, and we all know that oxygen is the secret of good health.

Cabbage will also help significantly in ulcer cases. The healing essential oils in the cabbage bring healing to the inner lining of the stomach through the kaolin. Cabbage is rich in this mineral, and the soft tissue of the stomach regenerates its lining through its properties.

Cabbage salads are simply a terrific, rich source for enhancing the immune system.

If you only choose one vegetable to eat daily, let it be cabbage, and your nutrition would be complete, beautifully balanced and sufficient.

Carrots

We grew up honestly believing that carrots were good for your eyes, because bunnies do not wear glasses. I know it seems a bit silly now, but the vision benefits from carrots are no joke. Fresh carrots are healthy for so many reasons. It is very rich in vitamin A, which is vital in good vision. Since everything in our body is connected the eyes are not independent entities either. Our eyes are dependent upon our overall health. Unfortunately, children and adults with diabetes are living proof to that truth. We need to remember that everything we allow our children to put into their mouth should be only to serve their health. Junk food is as it sounds; Junk, or garbage, you decide.

Giggling Dr. Green

Healthy food provides all the building bricks the child (as well as yourself) needs for optimum development.

Carrots are known in the natural therapy world, as "A major enemy to cancer". Knowing about the phytochemicals and the antioxidants helps us understand why the carrot is such a valuable cancer fighter. Carrot juice, combined with celery and beets, can take us from seriously sick, to very healthy. It is nature's chemotherapy in a very colorful and tasty elixir of life.

Carrots are also not very appreciated by the many parasites residing in one's intestines and blood.

Many children suffer from different types of worms and other parasites, and the allopathic medications offered are like all medications, with harmful side effects. However, carrot juice, or just ground carrots with a tiny little bit of garlic, have only a harmful side effect on the worms and parasites, not on the child.

Celery

Celery can be used in fresh raw salads and is a healthy tasty crunchy snack. The celery is probably the richest in fiber, and kids enjoy the juiciness of it. It recommends fresh, raw, and organic only and does not use the commercialized dips. Make your own healthy dip.

Cucumber

Cucumber is the favorite vegetable for many children. Even though it seems like nothing but water, it still is an important food in every fresh vegetable salad. The minerals, vitamins and fiber of the cucumber are worth the little effort it takes to prepare. The best cucumbers are …you guessed it, from the Middle East. They are smaller than the English cucumbers and the American cucumbers and taste better; they are grown in California as well. You can grow them in your own little patio or balcony even in a flowerpot. Enjoy; they are healthy for every child and parent. Please make sure to get the organic cucumbers only.

Garlic

Nature's best antibiotic.

Rich in minerals and essential oils.

A proven cancer-preventing ingredient. Helps fight colds, and when prepared with brown sugar or molasses, relieves colds and congestions.

Helps to heal and relieve the pain from wasp stings when applied to the skin.

Giggling Dr. Green

When served first thing in the morning helps small children with worms.

Helps to prevent ameba and other parasites.

Garlic is so rich in its healing assets, that it would be wise to read more about it specifically.

Kale

Kale is vital for the immune system for its chlorophyll which improves blood consistency and the ability to bind with more oxygen. The red blood cells are enriched by kale. Kale is rich in iron and calcium, and is overall a very healthy food and is recommended as highly as broccoli and perhaps even more.

Onion

Slice a raw onion and pour brown or raw sugar on top, then let it sit for an hour or two, and serve the syrup to your child in cases of severe cough and colds. Opens any congestion, and helps for sinus infections, also, like garlic, onions is a natural antibiotic. Rich in minerals and vitamins, like magnesium we all need for our stable health, vitamin be, Kaolin, etc. If your child is sick and you place an onion at his bedside, the next morning your child will be well.

Good to use for mosquito bites, bees, wasp and even scorpion and spider bites when applied on the skin.

Raw onions are very helpful for allergies and hay fever.

Best part in every salad, and the best appetite opener in the kitchen. You can never have a good kitchen without onions.

Parsley

Parsley is good for bladder infections, burning urine, skin rash, eczema, pink eye water retention, swellings and edema and more. Parsley will contribute to healing low hemoglobin as spinach does due its chlorophyll and high iron content. Parsley is rich in iron, and calcium.

In cases of bladder infections, high blood pressure and edema, the best way to treat it naturally with parsley is; pouring boiling water into a glass with fresh parsley, let it stir for a few minutes, and drink. It helps; it has no harmful side effects, and is inexpensive.

Wonderful enriching spice for every raw or cooked dish.

Potatoes

Giggling Dr. Green

The most familiar potato dish to American children is French fries. Little do they know that this is not the only way to enjoy this divine vegetable. Potatoes have enormous healing assets.

Potato juice heals ulcers, and many stomach complaints. It is a secret we don't hear from the doctors since not much money is involved in this age-old medicine.

When you need to heal an ulcer, which is usually diagnosed in the stomach, you can just juice a raw potato, drink it on an empty stomach and within just a few days you can actually free yourself of this painful disorder.

What makes it so healing? Simple; potatoes are rich in kaolin, (like cabbage) as well as many other minerals. All these are emitted together with the very delicate starch of the raw potato. I remember how our parents would apply potato starch on our itching wounds when we were little.

Cough. Here is another good way to apply potatoes for your health, and is part of our homemade pharmacy.

When the child is coughing and struggling with chest pain, cook the potatoes and mash them. When the mass is still nicely warm, NOT HOT, mound the potato mash on a towel, fold it to the size of the child's chest, and let it lay on the chest, or the back for as long as it stays warm. It will ease the chest pain, and calm the cough. It keeps it nice and warm, without the hazards of an electric pillow.

In general, potatoes contribute significantly to our child's health provided they are not fried in any way, and please; cook and serve them unpeeled. Potatoes have to be cooked in their skin in order for us to receive the full health benefits from all the treasures they hold.

Never eat a potato that starts to become green. It is toxic.

Romaine Lettuce

The whole point in green leafy vegetables is that they are green. Green means rich in iron and so rich in oxygen - the traditional natural health says, "Green makes red". Green leaves help to create hemoglobin. It is absolutely vital for good health and a strong immune system. Iceberg lettuce, in my opinion, is a "waste of space on the plate and in the stomach". It is pale and lifeless. The

Giggling Dr. Green

greener the better. The romaine lettuce is very juicy and can be consumed just as is even without any spices or dressing.

Snow peas and sugar snaps

Snow peas and sugar snaps are renowned for their health assets. They are considered as very dangerous….to cancer cells.

Dr. Heimann, from Netherland, treated his cancer sick patients with snow peas and sugar snaps and his results were of amazing success rate. They are an absolutely delicious and healthy snack.

No sugar and no fat. Just munch on them raw and get well.

Giggling Dr. Green

Spinach

Kids can just munch on young spinach leaves with their little hands and never be anemic again. Spinach is THE blood cleaner and immune system booster.

Rich in calcium, iron, vitamins and minerals, and, of course, chlorophyll. Spinach is the most "Light through food" supplier we have. Remember –cells filled with light are happy and healthy. Spinach helps to strengthen us when recovering from any illness. Eat lots of spinach to help overcome lingering fatigue.

Sweet potatoes

What a delicious way to enhance vitamin A consumption. There are so many different ways to prepare them, and the health benefits are impressive.

My friend prepared for her son 5 cups of fresh squeezed juice made of carrots, celery, beets, kale and fresh sweet potato. Within 2 weeks, his tumor disappeared and it took just 2 more weeks for him to resume a normal life. Sweet potatoes contain kaolin which is a health improving mineral for the inner lining of the digestive system.

Tomato

These are somewhat controversial in the healing arts. Tomatoes are acidic and not always tolerated by everyone. Even though their healing qualities are obvious, they still need to be eaten with discernment. For instance, people who suffer from kidney problems should not eat tomatoes. However, tomatoes are indispensable for their high content of vitamin C, and many other vitamins and minerals. The only real problem is that we must look for those that are not genetically engineered, and that ripened on the vine and do not come from the greenhouse. The only really healthy tomatoes are the natural grown ones that were picked when ripe. The rest are unhealthy. Everyone should have a spot on their balcony or porch devoted to growing tomatoes in a container, so they can be enjoyed at the peak of redness.

Grains, Nuts and Seeds

Almonds

No need to worry about calcium, Omega 3, or about getting enough iron and protein into our child's diet - when he gets just a fist full of almonds a day, or a fresh glass of almond milk for him. Almonds supply more calcium than any dairy product. Just 10 almonds give more calcium than 1 glass of milk, And - have absolutely none of the harmful side effects that milk has.

Giggling Dr. Green

When children suffer from digestive problems, allergies, heartburn, weakness, almonds, almond milk or almond spread will help. Raw almonds are always the best choice

Best almond cheese is easy to prepare and is an excellent source of probiotic on top of all the many benefits we have in almonds.

Brown Rice

Brown rice supports healthy bones, hair, and is easy for digestion with plenty of fiber.

Prevents bone loss and fortifies the immune system.

Rich in B vitamins and E.

Cooked rice alleviates upset stomach and diarrhea as the cooked brown rice water helps the healing process.

Good source of protein and carbohydrates.

Soothes the inner stomach and intestines linings, and helps in weight loss. Serves as a fine substitute for gluten and wheat intolerance, and preferred even if the gluten and wheat intolerance has not been diagnosed yet.

Chickpeas, beans and lentils

I would consider them as number one in plant protein providers.

The longer they cook the better they digest. Usually they make a whole protein when served with rice or quinoa or any other carbohydrates. Peas are whole proteins.

They are the perfect substitute for any animal derived protein, yet, do not have the side effects or damaging impact on the child's health, as the animal derived products have.

Traditionally it is the main dish in most of the cultures around the world, and the healthiest.

Flax Seeds

Vital in every nutrition as they help the digestive system inner linings, are anti-inflammatory and rich in omega 3, and 9. The soaked flax seeds soaked mucus, is one of the most anti-inflammatory assets we can ask from nature. Flax seeds are important for the neuronal tissue as well as brain fluid and cells. The flax seeds help prevent ulcers and constipations. For children with a tendency for hard stools, stomach aches, gas, constipation, internal inflammations, the flax seeds will serve as a regulator and enhance the child's self-healing ability. It is good to soak in water about an hour before use, or, to grind the seeds in a coffee grinder. The flax seeds have a nutty flavor and could be sprinkled on any food.

Fenugreek

Although not very popular and not very well-known in the Western Hemisphere, it is the most significant seed for good, stable and complete health. Fenugreek will help in building an excellent immune system. Regardless of how consumed, it is vital for our children as well as for us. In my small recipes suggestions chapter, I will share a few ideas for a very natural and simple way to use fenugreek.

Quinoa

Quinoa is an ancient Native American grain. Quinoa is very delicate and fine in its taste and structure. A very good source of protein, carbohydrates, calcium and iron.

Easy to cook and can be added to numerous dishes. Quinoa is also available in flour form, and is many times healthier for baking than wheat, or corn. You can also find quinoa in red, yellow, black and white.

Quinoa is an excellent substitute for grains and baking goods and because quinoa has no wheat and no gluten, it is absolutely safe for all.

Sesame seeds

Sesame seeds are very popular in the Middle and Far East cuisines. For some reason, the ancient cultures already knew about the importance of sesame. Sesame seeds are added to every pastry, breads, cakes, cookies, and their pressed oil enriches the Chinese and Japanese dishes. Sesame seeds are a good source of calcium and iron. The sesame seeds fat is rich in Omega 3 and . In my Israeli culture the sesame seeds are in Hummus, on the traditional Challah bread, cookies and many more dishes including breads, buns and salads. The healing and nutritional assets of the sesame seeds are indispensable.

For children with low calcium, iron and magnesium, I would highly recommend enriching the child's nutrition with these magnificent seeds.

It is a very healthy substitute and replacement for milk for kids as well as adults. If Americans were to use more of it, osteoporosis would probably be extremely rare.

Sunflower and Pumpkin seeds

Giggling Dr. Green

Like all seeds, sunflower and pumpkin seeds are rich in proteins, minerals and vitamins, fatty acids and are a must in every health oriented nutrition regime. They are whole nutrition and a tasty addition in every fresh vegetable salad, or when added to cooked rice or potatoes (add them raw only after cooking). They are rich in every nutrition ingredient we need, because they are seeds. Important for skin (raw!), for the brain and nerves. (Imagine, it is so good, healthy and nutritious and no one had to look into its sweet brown eyes and kill it for us to eat it)

Wild Oats (gluten free)

In Switzerland lived a very famous natural health practitioner whose name was Dr. Muesli.

I grew up on Muesli, which he claimed healed all his clients, young or old. Muesli is so easy to prepare, every child can do it.

My children use this simple recipe for their own children, whenever they decide to give them a little immune system boost.

Wild oats are known for their slimy texture once they are soaked in water. According to the Swiss tradition it is soothing and strengthening of the soft tissues. Natural Medicine has discovered that the inner linings of the stomach and the intestines are the major key for good health. The explanation is simple and makes a lot of sense; the stomach is an organ we digest and break down our food. The intestines are the part that transfers the nutrition into the body through the blood. When these organs function properly, the body can actually utilize and assimilate the nutrition and use it to nourish and keep the body alive and healthy. The next "station" would be the large intestines, to transport the waste out of the body. This too, if in order, keeps the body healthy and without any waste accumulation. If the large intestines work well, we have good evacuations and the health is well kept. Therefore, traditional natural medicine puts very high emphasis on the inner linings of the digestive system. We all know how sick and miserable a child can be if any of these organs are not well. Wild oats are known as skin soothing in case of any rash. Just blended in the bath water will calm any skin irritation.

Chia Seeds

Super food, rich in minerals and vitamins. Very nutritious as a protein supply. Can be used in all baking goods, salads, soups etc.

It can also be used instead of eggs

like the fax seeds.

Giggling Dr. Green

Mung beans

Like green peas are very rich in all necessary amino acids, besides the other nutrition properties. Very easy to digest.

I use it as flour in baking, and like them sprouted.

*These are just a few of the enormous varieties available as healthy nutrition supplies. It is very inexpensive yet very rich in all the nutrients we and our children need.

Herbs and spices

Anise

We can find anise fresh on the produce shelves, and eat it as a fresh salad, as well as using the seeds for health purposes. Anise seeds are part of herbal teas in cases of colds and coughs. Anise in its fresh form serves the blood cleansing and kidney stimulation. The respiratory system benefits from the healthy kidneys.

Chamomile

The flowers are small and daisy-like and have a sweet, apple-like flavor.

It is known for its properties of healing all inflammations and colds. It supports the body in its healing efforts and is considered in the healing arts to be the best natural antibiotic. When used as tea, chamomile helps to relieve any stomach discomfort, indigestion and gas. Since it is very potent, the tea must be prepared mild and be strained of the flowers after a few minutes. Never leave the flowers soaking too long because it makes the tea too strong, and may cause damage.

Chamomile is also very healthy for hair rinses after shampooing. Good for any skin and eye irritations as well. In the case of Red Eye for instance, take a chamomile tea bag, and make tea. Then take the cooled tea bag and lay it on the closed eye. It works wonders, is simple and cannot hurt.

It always works for colic for babies as well as stomach complaints in adults.

Flowers

There are many edible flowers. Not only do they garnish your plates and make it so beautiful and happy looking for the eyes, but also, they are very healthy when eaten. When children come to a table with the flowers on their plates, they are so happy their eyes light up. They feel as if the flowers are alive and "smiling" at them. The flowers have very delicate essential oils and tiny little phytohormones that will stimulate every vital function in the child's body. There cannot be anything more reviving, more re-vitalizing and more soothing to any child's mind, appetite and health condition than a beautiful flower on his/her plate that can actually even be eaten. Let your child eat the flower slowly. This way the wonderful feeling of the delicate flower and subtle sensual smells and the intricate parts of the flower will be soothing to your little guest for dinner. Your child can learn to be so attentive to the fine flower smell and how it connects to the taste buds. It is so very relaxing and healing, like eating by candlelight with soft music, so soothing. Treat your children as if they are fine company in your home, for truly they are. They are ours to nurture for such a short time, and the things we teach them will then transfer to the way our grandchildren will be raised. So please, set lovely, peaceful meals, and make your children feel as though they are your honored vip guests.

Some of the edible flowers are Dandelions, Orchids, Pansies, Carnations, Jasmine, and Roses.

Stevia

A small beautiful white flower and a very sweet bush, not only to the observing eye but also in its taste. If you clip a leaf off the bush and taste it, you will find it very sweet. Stevia is a healing herb and known to lower cholesterol. In drops or powder, it serves as a healthy sweetener and is able to be used as a substitute in every sweet dish preparation as well as a sweetener for beverages such as tea, lemonades, best in hot drinks. Use it scarcely for it has a profound taste slightly on the bitter side.

Thyme

Thyme is a healthy spicing herb with plenty of healing properties. Thyme has been known for hundreds and perhaps thousands of years. There are many different types of thyme and many different uses.

In the Middle East, it is used as a spice in many different dishes. Thyme is used for all kinds of stomach ache complaints such as skin complaints, kidney issues, headaches, colds etc. Finely chopped and mixed with sesame seeds, sea salt and olive oil is a delicious dip for pita bread, buns or just topping the salad, the way the traditional Mediterranean folk use it. Thyme is a healthy and tasty natural spice with a delicious taste.

Turmeric

Giggling Dr. Green

Not only adds a nice yellow color to the rice, or any dish you cool, but is very healthy to the immune system. It is known in the Middle Eastern diet as an important spice for most dishes.

A healing spice.

- These are just a few of the vast herbs and spices at our disposal to enrich our dishes to better taste and health promotion

Apple Cider Vinegar

Does not sound very yummy but is the best medicine in your natural first aid kit. Apple Cider Vinegar (ACV) is an old traditional medical asset. The Far Eastern nations also use Rice Vinegar, and Persimmon Vinegar. In East and Western Europe, the ACV has been the trend for eons. Yet, had it been just a trend, it would not be researched and kept for so many generations as the ACV has been. ACV has many uses, as a healing product as well as a strengthening and prevention asset.

Healthy Food = Healthy Children

Here are a few very simple suggestions to prepare some of those foods to help your children achieve and maintain optimum health.

Brown Rice

Baby's First Cereal

For small babies, as young as 3 months old, brown rice should be powdered in a coffee grinder. For 2 TBLS of the rice powder add 1-cup of water and cook for at least 25-30 minutes, stirring often. The cereal will be very smooth and easy to digest for the baby.

If you are a little creative, you can add freshly grinded quinoa and buckwheat to the pot.

Himalayan salt and a little olive or good coconut oil will delight it even more and your baby will gobble it down - and thrive.

Adding steamed vegetables - wow, what a healthy feast.

Cereal for toddlers and up

For older children just as you would cook white rice, just add ½ cup more water for each cup of rice. Adding a few raisins or one chopped date would be very welcome to most children, and increase the nutritional value. (The same can be prepared using Quinoa, amaranth, millet, gluten free wild oats etc.)

Giggling Dr. Green

Try serving with cinnamon and a grind apple, or a squeezed Clementine's and your children of all ages will clean their bowls every time!

Soaked brown rice for an hour before cooking opens the grains up and it cooks faster. Try adding a little wheat free Tamari Sauce or Bragg to the lunch or dinner serving; the taste is delicious.

A thoroughly cooked brown rice serves well for intestinal disorders. It has the same soothing elements as gluten free wild oats, and is traditionally used in natural medicine since it helps the inner stomach linings to heal quickly.

There is no need to worry about constipation, since brown rice has plenty of fiber and bran that keeps the bowels moving properly and comfortably.

Roasted Rice

When I was a child, I loved the brown rice roasted slightly in a dry pan, and when it started to pop, we would very slowly and carefully add the boiling water, then turn the heat down to very low, cover the pan, and let it simmer for 20-30 minutes. This was the very best rice I ever ate.

With Almonds and Raisins

In many different cuisine traditions, there are various add-ins for the rice. For instance, you can add peeled almonds, and raisins to the cooking rice. This makes a very elegant and delicious rice to serve as a meal in itself or as a wonderful side dish.

Brown Rice and Onions

You can add lightly roasted sliced onions, a little chopped dill, cumin powder, sea salt and a spoon of Extra Virgin Cold Pressed Organic Olive Oil to your cooked brown rice. You will love it forever and so will your children.

Brown Rice Patties

Brown rice can be precooked and then mixed with flax seeds or chia seeds, replacing eggs form into little patties and fried on a cast iron pan with just a light spray of Pam, or baked. This will please the children who like to hold the food in their hands, and like it a little firm rather than puree. Please do not forget to spice them. Spices stimulate the digestive enzymes secrets and are very healthy, if natural.

Brown rice salad or (quinoa, buckwheat)

Brown rice makes delicious cold salads for hot days.

Giggling Dr. Green

When children return from school and have no desire for a warm meal in the summer, the precooked brown rice can be tossed and mixed with chopped bell peppers, chopped red onions, one spoon of extra virgin cold pressed Olive Oil, a dash of fresh ground white pepper, chopped cilantro, pumpkin seeds and a lemon juice. You can add as many other veggies as you please. Let your culinary imagination run wild. A visit to the fresh farmer's market will inspire you to toss in the freshest seasonal produce and will be a delight for both the eyes and mouth. The children will love it, and you will be happy to know that your kids just had a complete meal with all the necessary ingredients. No meat is necessary. Brown rice is rich in good protein, and meat is an unwanted, unnecessary and unneeded addition. I personally would never serve a child meat, because it is so unhealthy and known for causing the worst diseases.

Please keep in mind that brown, red, wild or any kind of unbleached and unprocessed rice is a whole nutrition for itself. Children who grow up on natural rice have no nutritional deficiencies of any kind. Therefore, every time you prepare any kind of unprocessed rice you add a significant enhancement to your child's health and development.

- I grind the rice in either the coffee grinder or my vita mix and use the flour to bake the best cookies for my family.

Avocado - spicy or sweet

Avocado can be prepared more on the spicy side or on the sweet and sour side.

Avocado has to be ripe in order to have all the benefits necessary.

Spread or Dip

To make a delicious spread, all you need is - half a fresh lemon squeezed to the peeled and mashed avocado. Lemon keeps the avocado from getting brown while adding flavor and health benefits. Add some chopped onion, green, red or white makes no difference, fresh ground white pepper and a small bit of sea or Himalayan salt. Mix thoroughly and you have a wonderful and healthy spread. It is served with a bowl of fresh celery and carrots as a dip. I do not know any child who does not enjoy it. If you blend the mixture for a minute in the blender, it will give it a very smooth texture.

Avocado salad

With a melon ball spoon, scoop small mounds out of the avocado.

Add chopped onion, small pieces of orange, chopped pieces of romaine lettuce, peeled almonds, a little bit of sea or Himalayan salt, 1 tbsp extra virgin cold pressed organic olive oil, and plenty of fresh squeezed lemon juice. This one will have you planting avocado trees in your backyard!

Avocado with Tofu

Blend the avocado with silk extra firm tofu, adding 1 fresh squeezed lemon, sea or Himalayan salt and little fresh ground white pepper. This delightful creamy blend can be used as the foundation for so many wonderful recipes. Be as creative as you like! Use your family's favorite seasonings and additions.

Avocado spreads are so versatile, by changing the mix-ins, you can create endless delicious dishes for your families' health and pleasure.

Guacamole

This dip or spread is delicious and nutritious as well. Use ripe, mashed avocado, cilantro, chopped onion and a fresh jalapeño pepper, finely diced, along with Himalayan salt and fresh ground white pepper. Some people add chopped tomatoes to their guacamole, also and it takes on extra nutrients, texture and flavor when mixed in. I like to make the guacamole without the tomatoes, and then serve it on top of thick slices of tomatoes. Very pretty on the dish, fun to eat and very healthy for your family. If you place a ripe black olive on top of the guacamole after you mount some onto the tomato slice, your children will think it is a party!

Avocado with Sauerkraut

My dear friend Valerie introduced me to another very healthy avocado dish.

Take a ripe avocado, peel it and give a couple of whirls in the blender or mash it up. Add salsa (with no additives) and sauerkraut. This makes a delicious dip for all ages. The sauerkraut is known for its vitamin B12 production in the intestines and so a PH balance, which enhances oxygen utilization and absorption.

Avocado Cream

When I was a little girl my aunt knew how much I loved her avocado cream. Her recipe is simple and soothing. The kind of memory that makes you smile and as an adult you want your children to experience it too. Take well-mashed avocado, a little honey or maple syrup, lemon and cinnamon powder and blend them real good in a food processor. What a nice creamy dessert that is well tolerated by nearly everyone. If after you mix it well you mount it into a pretty bowl and decorate it with mandarin slices. A real treat.

Asparagus

The simplest way is to steam it for a few minutes. This vegetable promotes kidney health, is tasty and refreshing. Can be seasoned with a pinch of

Giggling Dr. Green

Himalayan or celtic salt, fresh squeezed lemon juice, extra virgin cold pressed olive oil, and chopped parsley and garli

c and balsamic vinegar after asparagus has slightly cooled. For a pretty garnish, I would toss some chopped dill on top and some lightly roasted pine nuts.

String Beans

Like asparagus, string beans are kidney stimulants and are an ancient "prescription" for even healing them. Since it is not a medication they can be served to our children without boundaries.

All string beans need to be washed, the tough ends snapped off, steamed in little water. After steaming, strain and let them cool off. Add fresh squeezed lemon, crushed fresh garlic, a little sea or Himalayan salt, chopped fresh dill, rosemary and a spoon of extra virgin cold pressed olive oil. Very tasty and satisfying.

In general, put very little water in the pot when steaming any vegetable. If there is any water left in the pot after steaming, pour it in a container, continually add and store in your fridge after a few days you will have enough of this vegetable extracted water to start a wonderful soup stock. The water holds the essence of vitamins and minerals that were in the vegetables, and we sure don't want to toss them out. True energy water, healthy and can be used to cook your rice in, or soup.

Fenugreek dish

Fenugreek is an ancient, well-known remedy and is a valuable preventative for better health and fitness for our families.

Serves as a blood purifier and stimulates the immune system for all ages. It is perhaps the best anti-inflammatory food.

Here is a great recipe I picked up from a wonderful Yemen friend from Israel.

Ingredients

3 Tsp of fresh ground fenugreek seeds

½ cup fresh squeezed lemon juice

2-4 garlic cloves, minced

1 tbsp extra virgin cold pressed olive oil

1 medium sized tomato, coarsely chopped

½ tsp Himalayan or sea salt

1/4 tsp chili pepper

Giggling Dr. Green

1 tsp thyme

½ bundle fresh cilantro, chopped

1-2 cup water

Grind the seeds well when they are still dry.

Soak the ground seeds in room temperature water overnight.

The next morning, rinse gently.

(If you do not rinse, the fenugreek is healthier, yet a little bitter).

Blend with garlic and water, (Do not cook or even warm up. It is raw and should stay that way!)

Add the lemon, sea salt, tomato, thyme, chili pepper, and olive oil, mix well.

Fenugreek Sprouts

Soak seeds in a full glass of water, overnight.

Put the soaked seeds in a jelly jar and cover the jar with a piece of gauze or cheesecloth.

Turn the jar upside down and let it rest in a shaded, well-aired place. Continue to rinse it well two or three times a day. It is important to keep the seeds well rinsed, with no water remaining. The seeds need to be kept moist, but not in standing water. Let the sprouts grow to the size you like.

The sprouts are not only delicious and crunchy in salads, and just eaten out of hand, but they are an important health promoting asset. Here our children can learn how to sprout, and have them grow their own delicious healthy food. You can sprout any seeds keeping in mind they are the most potent and powerful nutrition.

Cabbage

Cabbage also holds ancient traditional, medicinal magic for numerous health needs, as well as for prevention benefits. Many books have been published about the medical assets the green as well as red cabbage contains. The best and easiest way to digest cabbage is in its fresh, raw state. It is a myth that cabbage is hard to digest. However, if it is for you, it is only because you have to eat it raw to heal your digestive tract.

Cabbage Salad

Ingredients:

Giggling Dr. Green

1/2 head white cabbage

3 fresh carrots

3 celery stalks

3 tbsp rice vinegar/Kombucha

2 tbsp apple cider vinegar

1 tsp sea or Himalayan salt

½ tsp fresh ground white pepper

2 tbsp extra virgin cold pressed olive oil

Some minced garlic and fresh chopped thyme can be added if you would like a more Middle Eastern flavor to it.

1-2 squeezed lemons

1 tsp Caraway seeds

1/2 Cauliflower

Chop the vegetables as fine as you like them.

(I like salads very finely chopped, whereas my husband prefers the coarser chunks of carrots and celery, and more of a shredded cabbage. Lucky for him, he makes the salads in our home!)

Add the garlic and thyme now, if you are using them, and season with the salt, pepper, vinegars and olive oil.

Let it stay in the bowl for ½ hour and toss it well before refrigerating.

The biggest benefit of this salad, besides its health assets, is; the longer it stays the better it gets.

Homemade Original Humus

Ingredients

½ cup garbanzo beans (soaked overnight in water and cooked until very soft)

Juice from a fresh squeezed lemon

2 tbsp raw Tahini (raw ground slightly roasted sesame seeds)

1/2 tsp sea/ Himalayan salt

1 cup of water

2-3 garlic cloves

1-2 tbsp extra virgin cold pressed olive oil

Giggling Dr. Green

Blend all ingredients beginning with ½ the cup of water. Continue adding water until a nice creamy texture is achieved.

Taste, if it seems to be missing something, adding more lemon will nearly always do the trick. (Be sure to have the garbanzo beans cooled off completely before preparation)

The best way to eat it is to spread on gluten free pita, rice cakes, or, dip, or even raw small carrots, cucumbers and any other bite-sized vegetables, or serve with a nice Middle Eastern vegetable Salad.

Typical Middle Eastern Salad

Here is how you prepare it:

1 large tomato

1 cucumber

1 bell pepper

1 medium onion

¼ bundle fresh parsley

Fresh cilantro

Lemon, sea/ Himalayan salt, a little fresh ground black pepper, extra virgin cold pressed olive oil.

Cut the vegetables, add the seasonings and toss well.

Basic mediterranean Salad

Children love this salad because they can just dig in and choose from all the different colors and flavors. Despite this salad's name, please do not save it for only special dinners. Any meal you serve will seem special, and your children are the finest company you will ever entertain.

1 carrot

5 or 6 sugar snap peas

5 or 6 cherry tomatoes

5 or 6 fresh mint leaves

4 fresh romaine lettuce leaves

1 red bell pepper

A fist full of baby spinach fresh leaves

¼ red onions

Giggling Dr. Green

1 fresh lemon

1 tbsp raw pumpkin seeds

1 tbsp raw sunflower seeds

1 small Middle Eastern cucumber (the small, slim cucumbers)

¼ grated lemon peel

1 tbsp extra virgin cold pressed organic olive oil

¼ tsp sea /Himalayan salt

¼ avocado

1 tbsp Apple Cider Vinegar/Kombucha

Cut all the vegetables into 1" sized pieces. Wash lemon, and then peel half of it. Cut the lemon half into very small pieces. Squeeze the other half of the lemon into the salad. Add the oil seasons and salt. Toss well - enjoy.

Remember to wash the vegetables thoroughly before preparation.

Non-Dairy Cream Cheese (Can be prepared from homemade almond yogurt too)

Ingredients

1 package Silken Tofu extra firm

1 medium sized Fresh lemon –juiced

¼ teaspoon sea salt

If you roll the unpeeled, uncut lemon before juicing, you will get much more juice out of it.

Place the ingredients in a blender, and whirl on high for 1 minute.

Any seasoning can be added to this basic non-dairy cream cheese.

Adding some chopped chives and a bit of fresh ground pepper makes a quick dip for celery stalks.

A little ground cinnamon and a few raisins mixed into the basic spread would be a very nice dip to eat with apple wedges or top a vegan cheesecake.

Be creative, this is such a versatile basic spread, unlimited to what you can create with it.

Notice:

Giggling Dr. Green

Soy and tofu are very rich in calcium, iron and omega fats. It is the best available protein for us which doesn't leave the harmful by-products that dairy and meat do leave. It is a safe and very nutritious food with countless variety options for preparation. Please do not listen to those who doubt the value of soy due to their own ignorance and the meat dairy industry propaganda for their own pocket. Tofu is so rich in digestible and easily assimilated protein that one serving is equal to a huge steak, yet, doesn't have to be killed, does not come with liver cancer producing side effects, does not clog the arteries, and has simply no down sides. Yes, it is white and not red, and also doesn't need the preservative Como flush.

Rolled gluten free Wild Oats Power Bars

(Not for very sensitive gluten intolerant individuals)

Ingredients

4 cups gluten free raw wild oats

1 cup rice flour (or any gluten free healthy whole flour)

½ cup unsweetened coconut flakes

½ cup organic raisins

1 tsp aluminum free baking powder

1 cup almonds (for young children it would be best to grind the almonds)

1 tsp vanilla extract (natural)

1 orange and one green apple diced and pureed

2 tbsp honey of maple syrup (organic fresh)

1 cup dried, chopped apricots (unsulfured)

1 cup dates cut in small pieces.

1 tbsp flaxseed or chia seeds with 3 tbsp water (let it rest for a couple of minute and then beat like you did eggs)

1 tbsp Unsulfured Molasses

1/2 tsp sea /Himalayan salt

½ tsp Cinnamon

Mix all the ingredients until the entire mixture is moistened.

Roll into small sized balls (golf ball size) and place on a cookie sheet, on waxed paper. Place in a preheated, 350° oven for 20 minutes.

Giggling Dr. Green

Gluten, Dairy and Egg-Free waffle

Ingredients

Let it all rest for an hour.2 cups of gluten free all-purpose flour. (You can just use rice flour mixed with Tapioca flour, garbanzo beans flour, soy flour, teff flour or corn flour)

1 ¼ cups of rice/almond/sesame milk or water/juice

2 tbsp raw honey of maple syrup

1 tsp aluminum free baking powder

½ ripe Avocado

3 tbsp flax seeds with 9 tbsp water (eggs substitute)

1/3 cup organic raisins

1/8 cup raw organic pumpkin seeds

1/8 cup raw chia seeds

Mix all the fluids together and add the flour and baking powder mix gradually, until well mixed. Do not over mix. Add the seeds and raisins.

Preheat the waffle iron and pour the batter on ¾ of the pan.

Allow to cook until steam is no longer visible.

Lemonade

In a glass of water add 1-2 tsp maple syrup (organic). Add lemon, ginger, a cinnamon stick, a few mint leaves if desired. Give children something good to drink other than soda with harmful artificial ingredients. Spend some time listening to the child, as he sips his lovely elixir, and perhaps you will hear the real reason behind his blues.

Banana Smoothie

Blend 2 cups of rice, oat or almond milk, one ripe banana, a few drops of pure vanilla essence, blend quickly for 90 seconds. For a frozen treat, add frozen strawberry, and some black berries, or orange juice.

After blending, pour this into small cups, and stick a small spoon in each cup. When frozen, pop one out for your child, and be prepared to be asked to make those often.

Frozen Grapes

Giggling Dr. Green

Wash thoroughly and dry. Put the grapes in the freezer and serve as a nice summer healthy cold snack. Careful! It is too good!

Best and healthiest Muesli

I prepare the dry mix so it will be easy and available even when I am short of time.

Exact portions are irrelevant.

Mix:

Gluten free wild oats

Hemp seed hearts

Pumpkin seeds

Sunflower seeds

Goji berries

Raisins

Flax-seeds

Chia seeds

Nutritional yeast flax

Chopped nuts (any)

Chopped dried apricots

Keep the mix dry until you need it.

When preparing the muesli:

Take about 3 tbsp of the mix per person. Let it soak in water covering it only for an hour or overnight

Add any fruit juice, any cut and/or blended fruit

Add 1 tbsp raw honey - or customize

A Swiss originated dish for the entire family's good health.

A few more tips;

- Learn to make homemade Kombucha. It is a vital pro-biotic and can be used as drinks, added to salads, mixed with juice, etc. It is a whole pharmacy worth owning in your home pharmacy kit.

Giggling Dr. Green

- Homemade chocolate is extremely easy to make with maple syrup instead of sugar, without any emulsifiers and dairy free, and is actually a very healthy asset.
- Ferment as many different vegetables as you like. Unlike the purchased canned pickles, your homemade will have what they are intended to have - probiotic agents.
- Make your own falafel mix, gluten free and with only the best chosen ingredients. Instead of deep-frying, rather make small muffins of it in your oven. So much healthier and delicious, and not fattening.
- Make your own cookies with natural ingredients like organic vanilla, maple syrup, and green ground apple instead of oil, use coconut oil if necessary instead of any other vegetable oil, use flax seeds rather than eggs, and add plenty of gluten free wild oats to any recipe.
- Almond milk is easy to prepare, leaving it on the counter overnight will make a good yogurt and then hanging it in a cheese cloth makes a base for best cheese.
- Nutritional yeast, flax seeds, chia seeds, hemp seeds, pumpkin seeds, all nuts and almonds and all seeds are best if organic, and kept in tight containers in the freezer. Are a must have in every kitchen

Gluten free and vegan lifestyle

Gluten and dairy are food components in almost all western diets. They are also one of the most significant reasons for so much disease and ailments. Gluten sensitivity is not detected just by diarrhea and intestinal bleedings, but through many different allergies. If your child's doctor does not find the allergy cause, I urge you to try eliminating all gluten from your child's diet for a few months. In at least 98% of the cases, there will be a marked increase in the child's health, as you discover his intolerance - to gluten.

That fact certainly will alarm many Western parents, since we see it as an impossible mission to maintain a gluten free diet for our children. If your child is allergic to gluten the odds are very good that one or both of you parents is allergic to wheat and gluten. Many cancers, ulcers, arthritis, skin problems, and even autism have been associated with gluten intolerance. Imagine, if the gluten and wheat is digested in the mouth, and the little children eat without their teeth, or they cannot chew yet, or, they are fast eaters, the chance that the gluten and wheat will be broken down is slim, to say the least. In order to digest gluten and wheat, we have to get used, from early on to keep the food for as long as possible in the mouth. This is in order for the enzymes in the saliva to actually start the initial process of the wheat and gluten digestion. How many adults keep bites of cake or of a sandwich in their mouths for any length of time, let alone children? The only chance the body can break down the gluten and wheat in order for the body to digest and assimilate it as nutrition - would be in the mouth, providing - your body produces those enzymes in the first place.

In the intestine, since we have no enzymes to digest the wheat and gluten will stay and ferment. This will create gas and pain. When this process repeats itself as often as it does in the average western diet it turns into toxins the body cannot release. The child may then develop all kinds of complaints, that may not actually and clearly point to the wheat and gluten yet, may be displayed as asthma, ADD, ADHD, cancer, tonsillitis, chrons, colitis, anemia, eczema, Autism, allergies, joint pain, constipation, diarrhea, or even as skin problems, and the list is endless. It is not easy to detect the correlation between the gluten and wheat intolerance with the different health disorders and the child may remain with his or her unresolved unhealthy condition for as long as the wheat and gluten continues to be in the diet. It took me many years to discover it yet, since I stay away from all, but literally all, gluten and wheat containing foods, I enjoy wonderful, steady and consistent good health. My children are sensitive to gluten and wheat but continue to disregard it. When trying to fight health problems, besides emotions, which I think should be addressed first; I would then search for the problem caused by the diet. It is the most common reason after the emotions. However, to suppress these sensitivities with allergy shots, or skin ointments and constipation medicines etc, will never restore health. The body will have to continue and expel the toxic elements that are supplied on regular bases into its system. This is nothing short of a struggle for survival in spite of the wrong treatments.

The important fact you need to keep in mind is: gluten and dairy intolerance is NOT a disease and not even a disorder. It is completely natural and normal. The food industry has made it stand out, because we cannot eat all the produced junk out there that is a source of good income for the food industry as wheat is a very cheap product element. More cultures live without wheat and gluten rich products than those who do eat them. Yes, like any other toxin administered for all these years and creates symptoms that will alert against any further use. However, intolerance is not a disease or disorder. Please appreciate your child's reactions because it is his and her- lifesaver.

Since I am gluten free, I find that our nutrition has so much more variety than the "normal" diet. I also do not eat anything that had eyes, or anything that

Giggling Dr. Green

had a mother. I do not use dairy, and no processed food, and never use wheat or gluten products.

The big variety of wheat and gluten free grains includes:

Rice, Corn, Quinoa, Millet, Amaranth, Teff, buckwheat and more. They are all rich in protein, iron, calcium and good carbohydrates.

I make my own salad dressings, and believe me they taste like heaven. For baking, I use the same recipes you can find in most baking books, and make my own modifications. I use rice and almond, or coconut milk instead of cow milk. I use maple syrup, honey, banana or apple, dates, and raisins rather than sugar. I substitute eggs with flax seeds. I use avocado and/or applesauce, coconut oil, or green ground apple instead of butter, margarine or oil. I use tofu instead of cream cheese. I use fruit juice instead of milk as well. I use non-aluminum baking powder. My cakes and waffles are so tasty no one believes that they are healthy as well. There is endless information in libraries, websites from all over the world, for achieving and enjoying a gluten and dairy free diet. The only place I truly find it difficult to eat is in restaurants in the US and Europe. However, they are getting better and healthier as well. Statistics indicate that 1 out of 75 people are lactose and wheat intolerant. I personally think that all people should stay away from dairy, meat, eggs, wheat etc. because it is simply unhealthy for everyone. In my 60's I am healthy, flexible, slim, and free of any need for any medications. My nutrition is modest, simple and my main drinks are water and green or white tea.

My golden rule is, "Chop dinner, don't cook it". And also "Pick your food, don't kill it".

For many more delicious ideas for healthy food, I recommend getting the book "May All Be Fed", by John Robbins. You will be delighted with his recipes, and proud to serve your family in a delicious, nutritious way at every meal.

Water

Water is Life. Without water, no life can exist; and the same is true for you and me. To grasp how water influences our body, one must think of a plant. We are not far from the plants in our water consistency. Looking at a plant on a warm dry day, it is obvious how the leaves start to crumble, collapse and wither when the plant is losing too much water. Some plants close their leaves, and it seems as if the lawn, for instance, is changing color. This is the self-protection mechanism of the plant when threatened by dehydration. Waiting a little too long before "Saving" the plant, it simply dies. Except for most members of the cactus family that have adjusted to hot, dry, desert conditions, and therefore store water in its branches instead of leaves as they developed the thorns that do not lose as much water as regular fleshy leaves, all plants are dependent on receiving water frequently. Water is a matter of life and death for adults as well, even if they are not aware of it. Many heart attacks occur not necessarily because of heart disease, but simply because of dehydration and many could be prevented as the simplest remedy on earth is; cool, clear water.

The myth that young babies do not need to drink water, as many physicians advise mothers, is dangerous and as far from the truth as the east is from the west. Please, do not take your doctor's advice as scripture. Even if the doctor is a close family friend, or the wisest person you know, have some doubt, get second opinions, and educate yourself. This will always be the safest way to go especially when it concerns your child 's health.

Double the Trouble

When Iris first came to me with her baby twins, they were very weak and sick. Their suffering was far too long and involved for their tender age of 6 months old. The fact that they were born slightly premature may have influenced their health a little, however the amounts of medications, hospitalizations, and wrong applications they had received, had placed those two little babies in serious danger. Thankfully, when they got out of the hospital their mother was completely fed up with their medical treatments, especially with the lack of encouraging results. One baby could not even cry because it was so hoarse, almost voiceless. Both had severe diaper rash, and the list of their ailments just went on and on. When addressing the hoarseness, Iris told me that the doctors had discovered a cyst on that child's vocal cords and decided to subject her to surgery soon. Needless to mention but it made me furious; surgery on this tiny baby for a cyst? After all, the very obvious reason for that cyst was the treatments the baby had endured in the hospital in the first place. The tube that was inserted into the child's tiny throat had injured the extremely sensitive tissue of the vocal cords and with the amounts of steroids this poor little girl received she developed a cyst. I was only surprised it was not both of the twins, since they had both endured similar treatments. Yet, the baby with the cyst was most likely injured while inserting the tube into her throat.

How did I know? The self-healing mechanism in the body heals such injuries naturally. The steroids are typically prescribed in order to "substitute" the hormones the body would derive from its own hormonal glands, in any injury.

Giggling Dr. Green

When treated with steroids, the injury "over-heels" so to speak in an imaginary description and creates the cyst. Cysts can heal by themselves very easily. All it needs is just a better circulation to the injured area. I could not believe my ears and Iris did not need more than to see the look on my face to understand my point. The diaper rash was so bad; I was not surprised at how that pain caused an ongoing restlessness and crying of both infants. The first thought that came to my mind was, Of course, *do they get enough water?* When I asked Iris, her response astonished me. She said; "The doctor said they don't need to drink water, they get a sufficient amount in their food". Do you drink water? I asked her. "Of course" was her prompt reply. So why don't these tiny babies deserve the same? I explained to her that infants have a greater need for water than adults, or even older children, since their bodies' water percentage is higher. Their bones are even not yet hardened and fully structured. Babies are dependent on water for their basic biological functions, all the time. They urinate often and their bowel movements are frequent, they perspire a lot, they cry, and their frequent movements. All these biological functions demand a very significant amount of water. If they do not receive sufficient water, they can get very sick; brain damage is even an option, as well as death. "But, Yael," she said, "Babies drink milk and get formula that has enough water in it, don't you agree? " I said; Blood consists of more than 85% of water. The kidney functions need the water; would you take a shower in milk or formula instead of water? Why do you think the kidneys should? Iris smiled and said, "So, why do you connect the skin rash with the water? The skin is not a kidney, and not the blood. ". The kidneys, I said, are responsible for the blood purification. If they are overwhelmed the lungs will have to help them to transfer the fluid impurities out of the body. The lungs will do that through the histamine by increased mucus production and the cough or runny nose will enable the baby to release the impurities and waste out of the body in order to maintain the balanced health. However, if the lungs are not developed enough yet, and like your babies, were treated with antibiotics and steroids in order to stop the mucus production, the body still has to deal with the waste removal. Therefore, if the lungs can't help the kidneys, the skin will have to carry the burden. The rash is the result of very acidic concentrated perspiration. Had the babies drank more water their kidneys would be able to remove the waste and the "help" from their lungs would not be needed. Yet, by administering the steroids, the lungs were "paralyzed" in a sense, and so the extremely concentrated waste fluids were sent to be flushed out through the capillaries. That caused the rash. So, I guess, the best way to remedy this rash would be, let the babies drink water.

Giggling Dr. Green

The very next day, Iris called happily to tell me both of the babies' rashes were all but gone. The baby cyst was not surgically removed and it disappeared as well shortly after we met. The secret: We are made of over 85% of water. It is a little humbling to consider ourselves in this light, however we truly are approximately 85% water and the rest is Bio-Electromagnetic field. Like the Quantum Physicists have claimed for many years already, there is the galaxy, then is the planet, then is the body, then is the molecules, then are the cells, then are the electrons and protons, then are the atoms, and then ... .is the energy. We consist of energy and even the water is energy. Water is even addressed in chemistry as H2O. Since that day Iris stopped seeing the doctor for her children and just made sure they had plenty of water, and the PEMF that helped her maintain good health for herself and her kids. I have been following the same regime for many years.

I never even go to bed without a bottle of water at my bedside. Often I see mothers struggling with a crying baby who seems inconsolable and unable to calm down. Neither the pacifier, food, toys, nor holding the baby would help. My suggestion is before you try to feed your baby and before you get worried and upset and before you try to feed your baby again, try water. This is what in many cases the first attempt should be. Imagine how on a hot day you walk through a long noisy and crowded mall, or on the street, or even in your own home, as suddenly you feel something is not feeling right to you. You just simply feel out of sync. You may feel irritable, anxious, weak, or even light headed. As if you ran out of energy. Would you take a pacifier to calm down? Would you be willing to have a bottle of formula be stuck into your mouth? Or being distracted with a noisy toy? Or, would you like to be rocked and hushed? I believe that a good glass of cold water could help you within seconds. So do your children. Water is also discharging the static magnetic field that is so harmful to our own natural healthy cells electromagnetic field, which charges us and the children in a public crowded place, a mall, or even in the car, Aircraft, train or theater.

When we feel irritable after being in a crowded and noisy public place for a while, we feel that we need something to calm this irritability down. Soothing your mind, body and spirit in water by showering or bathing would be the best choice. Relaxation in water is an ancient remedy whether in a Jacuzzi, tub, shower, glass of water, lake, sea, swimming pool, small pond or river. Water relaxes us naturally and is vital as it helps to discharge and rebalance our electromagnetic field. This will calm and balance the blood circulation, intestinal functions, brain activity, nervous system, skin, vitamin absorption, waste removal, fitness and overall well-being. We must have water inside and out at any time.

Giggling Dr. Green

Even our emotions are dependent upon water. Simply being near a water source is calming because water holds molecules of oxygen. So every environment close to water becomes enriched with oxygen. It is also loaded with negative ions. Negative ions are important for our health, because it is the opposite of polluted air. It means that the molecules in the air are loaded with oxygen instead of pollutants. The blood clotting that in the past was just of the old people's jargon sadly, is one of the many problems very young people suffer now a day as well. To address that problem in children as well as in adults, the best and least harmful way is to increase the daily water consumption.

It is our responsibility to help our children adopt the water drinking habit, often and abundantly. The best way to teach our children any healthy habit is by example. The MEGA force will tell you babies do not need water, and please turn our children into calves by forcing them to drink their milk at every meal. Forget it! Water and air are the only two elements you cannot go without for any length of time. Do you think it is a coincidence? Certainly not, the more and better fresh air and fresh water, the healthier your children will be and those are the least expensive medicines you can offer your children. Take your child on a hike and allow him to cup his hands and drink from a cool mountain stream. He will not be asking for soda that day only to return to that stream.

When we allow our children to pollute their growing bodies with sugared juice, soda, coffee, or the popular energy drinks such as Red Bull, coke, sprite, mountain dew etc. it is just like pouring poison into their cups, and that is the flat truth. Juices are only good if they are freshly prepared and served as a food substitute; it is not appropriate to serve any juice instead of water. Fruits and vegetables, which are composed of up to 95% water, are still not substitutes for drinking pure water. They are nutritious and the body does well handling them. The body gets its vitamins, minerals, fibers, proteins and carbohydrates. However, drinking water is vital for optimum health. We do not shower in grape juice, orange or lemonade. So, neither should the kidneys, the blood and heart. The more water we can consume and serve our children, the better their health potential becomes. When serving them soda or all the other kinds of liquids on the store shelves, we allow our children to become intoxicated with many harmful ingredients. Chemicals, toxic food colorings, artificially produced flavors, sugar in huge quantities, drugs, habit-forming additives, and more. None of these toxic and addictive chemicals are found in regular filtered and well-charged water. Since we are composed of 85% (and more) water, we must respect what we are made of and replenish it consistently. Our bodies are not made up of chemicals, white sugars, corn syrup, artificial colors or addictive substances, such as caffeine. So, as one of the key ingredients towards health for our children is to just help them to get used to enjoying water from the very first day, by serving this life elixir before trying anything else when they are cranky, crying, and restless and help them understand when they are a little older one day, the vital importance of water. We should really think of water as one of life's great pleasures and treasures, and it should be this way throughout our lives.

Chapter Three
Food without nutritional properties is poison

The supermarkets are filled to the brim with many different "new" foods. No wonder because stores must continue to grow. Unfortunately, many "new" foods are not edible and the majority of them, aside from having no nutritional value, actually set our children up for a lifetime illness. The food industry has turned into a careless and cold-blooded money making machine. Not even baby food is safe anymore. I do not mean to implant senseless paranoia in parents, however, please be discriminating and read the labels carefully, although even that is not always helpful. We better learn to read between the lines when it comes to commercialized food labels. Same as the wild animals protect their babies from harm's way and predators. I see the food industry as harmful as the drug industry; those two are like piranha forming an unholy alliance with vultures. The food industry is attacking our children at every turn, and the MEGA Force, being well represented in the pharmaceutical industry, comes along disguised as vultures, waiting to pick our pockets clean, as we desperately try to correct the damage all the new and improved foods have caused. Why would anyone put Melanin in babies' food? Had they been somewhat conscientious and responsible for the results of their products? Why does the dairy industry feed their livestock with hormones and medications they know very well would harm those who eat their products? Why would the meat industry put the dye into the meat on the display if they know how misleading and harmful they act? The meat color indicates the freshness however, if the meat is artificially colored we lose an important gauge for whether or not to eat what could be dangerously old meat; bad meat is deadly, (see the meat recall of over 20 million pounds of meat just September 2007, when the whole country was on alarm of life threatening bad meat supply). Deadly!

For my money, should I desire to ever buy a piece of a dead animal to eat, I would at least like to know if it was murdered recently*.

Giggling Dr. Green

King Solomon, said to be one of the wisest men to ever live, made the statement, "There is nothing new under the sun. If it is new, it isn't true, and if it is true, it isn't new." That applies perfectly to food. Vegetables, fruit, herbs, and freshwater have been available for our pleasure and proper health maintenance as long as recorded history, and beyond. Why would we want to buy sugared up chemicals, and deep fried artificial food products, when the world is abundant with nature's goodness? Do you suppose you are saving time and money when you buy a bag of potato chips instead of some fresh potatoes to prepare? Have you factored in the time and money sick children or having high cholesterol and heart disease will cost?

When you give your child a fruit flavored bag of processed snacks, have you considered the damage to his/her teeth you have just paid for? Eating an apple is exercise for the teeth, gums, jaw and facial muscles, however eating a gummed up bag of sugar not only sticks to the teeth like glue, but requires no effort, and therefore leads easily to overeating, tooth decay, gum inflammations, parasites in the intestines, etc. Junk food is a billion dollar industry; however look up the word **junk** in the dictionary. The Concise Oxford Dictionary's definition of "Junk" is "discarded articles, rubbish, anything regarded as having little value, a slang term for narcotic drugs". This seems to be an accurate description of the highly addictive, poisonous substances in the foods labeled as "junk food". Why should we feed our children and ourselves junk?

Do you offer your family these additives?

Aspartame

This sugar substitute is 200 times sweeter than sugar, and has been banned in baby food, it enhances the stimulatory effect of flavorings such as Monosodium Glutamate, and is known to adversely affect our nervous system and is a suspected carcinogenic (cancer causing agent).

Albumin

This is a component from the serum of animal blood

Ambergris

Secreted from the intestines of the sperm whale.

Arachidonic

This fatty acid is derived primarily from the liver, or brain of animals.

Caffeine

Giggling Dr. Green

An alkaloid that exists naturally in tea, kola nut and coffee; clearly toxic in high doses, can cause heart palpitations, high blood pressure, vomiting, convulsions, headache, diarrhea, frequent urination, dehydration, insomnia, stomach cramps, hand tremors, muscle twitches; acts as laxative, and as a bonus, it also saps the body's supply of calcium.

Would Pepsi, Coke and rest of the big players in the soda industry add addictive elements into their beverage if it did not serve their own purposes? As parents, we need to collectively call the foul as we see it and stop drinking soda ourselves.

Casein

A phosphor protein of milk which has a molecular structure that is extremely similar to that of gluten.

This is also used to make plastic, wow, a food that wraps itself after you eat it; you have to love that, right?

Catalase

This is derived from cow liver.

Monosodium Glutamate

This is an all-purpose seasoning used to enhance the flavors of food. It is a well-known neurotoxin (toxin affecting the brain) found in many snack foods, seasonings and take out foods.

Rennet

This cheese yeast is derived from calf stomach

Thimerosal

Used as a preservative this contains mercury and has been used in some vaccines and other products; FDA estimates that it is used in more than 30 licensed vaccines and biologics; the nervous system is very sensitive to all forms of mercury, methyl mercury and metal vapors are more harmful than other forms, exposure to high levels of metallic, inorganic or organic mercury can permanently damage the brain, kidneys and developing fetus, effects on brain functioning may result in irritability, shyness, tremors, changes in vision or hearing and memory problems

Torula

This is a high-protein additive, derived from wood sugars as a by-product of the pulping process in paper making; type S is used in baby food and cereals,

Giggling Dr. Green

type F is used in feed supplements for cattle, fish and chickens; toxic doses cause vomiting, diarrhea, restlessness, stomach irritation, depressed immune function and anemia.

Hmmm, what part of that last description makes me want to eat it or feed my baby with it?

Xylitol

A sugar substitute (bulk sweetener) found in some chewing gums. It is toxic to the brain, liver, and urinary passages in high doses and can cause diarrhea.

****

What does all this mean for our families health? It means that from a young age, our mentality, fertility, hormone levels, concentration levels, behavior, emotions, major organs of elimination, brain activity, and even our basic ability to learn and live holistically are all destroyed by mutated, heavily denatured processed foods and snack food products, all in the name of self-gratification and profits.

If you think these drugged up junk foods don't affect you, think again. All of the following can be attributed to their consumption: mental instability, by-polar, anxiety, irritability, depression, dental problems, dehydration, mucus, frequent colds, hyperactivity, Crohn's disease, impotence, unnatural cravings, diabetes, high blood pressures, kidney and liver problems, cancer, asthma, hair loss, bone loss, constipation, diarrhea, skin eruptions, foul smelling feces and urine, thrush, tiredness and even strong foot and body odor to name just a few. Surely, our children deserve better health. It is our responsibility to our kids' health and in order to prevent health problems later in life. Shouldn't we try to give them the best chance possible to be healthy and holistic in this polluted world? Will you run to pay their medical bills when they are 30 or 40 years old and can barely function without enough prescription medications daily to knock out an African Elephant?

Our sickness is big business; the MEGA Force cannot survive if we do not become ill, and so we cannot expect to get much help from them on our quest for health. Chemical producers sell their chemicals to food companies who in turn produce junk food. Food companies sell their products to consumers and in the process, advertising, marketing and packaging companies all get rich. Even the dentists benefit from most of the population having decayed teeth, plaque buildup and gum disease. This is not a conspiracy theory or an exaggeration of the true situation; these companies have absolutely no regard for our health. In fact, they have a vested interest in our continued dependency on their products, and the need for remedies from eating them. How many bottles of stomach ache relief medicine are sold because someone ate too much fresh salad, or soy products? May I suggest little or none! It is the fried, sugared, chemically enhanced and additive laden foods that send us running for relief in a bottle of pink chalky liquid, or a tablet of almost pure salt.

For the most part, chemicals approved for use in our foods by the Food & Drug Administration, MEGA Forces big brother, as it were, have never really had their effects tested on humans, and many countries even ban most of them. Scientists know the detrimental effects of the pesticides, preservatives and additives in our food contents. But once the foods have been exposed to large amounts of radiation, to kill germs and bacteria, then further refined, new mutant chemicals are created. When all combine together no one knows clearly the effects of those new substances on human health.

The younger the child, the easier it is to feed them naturally because they don't know the difference between mashed carrots, brown rice and broccoli with or without seasoning. Later on when they are grown they may continue to like it. Please do not enable or allow your children to become addicted to dangerous chemicals. Even your older children can still be favorably influenced, although it will take a bit of undoing. Be the example and show them the benefits in your own life. It really works. You can improve their diets by slowly replacing the offending foods. Find out which healthy ones they really like and let your children help you with shopping.

My suggestion is to stay completely away from all processed, pre packaged, cleverly disguised food products. (Was it you who went the extra mile to get the best service for your car, and got your Coke and Oriel cookies at the machine?) We care better for our car than for ourselves and our children's health. If the label boasts that it is "enriched with vitamins", do not touch it, unless you want to feed it to a pet you are tired of. I was kidding. The only way your baby or child can absorb and digest vitamins without harming their liver is by acquiring them naturally through healthy fresh food.

If the label reads, "modified food starches" do not touch unless you are trying to create a science project… These are very poisonous food preservatives. Corn Syrup is one of the worst products on the food market. If the FDA would do what they are paid for, they would take all those products with corn syrup off the shelves. Corn syrup is addictive and very damaging. The addition of corn syrup to most foods is probably responsible for many of the "epidemics" we find in children. Like diabetes, obesity, cancer, heart disease, hyperactivity disorders, kidney disorders and disease, liver problems in young children and so on. Any food product that includes that dreadful product should absolutely be banned in the responsible and health-conscientious home. This is filled with petroleum, and is absolutely harmful. Just because it helps your car run, do you really believe it fuels you well? I don't think so. Any food that the ingredient list includes words we cannot pronounce should not be touched.

Snacks such as potato chips, popcorn, fried pork skin, etc, should not be in your home, if you care for your child's health. Processed cheeses melted, cream cheese, mozzarella and all the rest, should never be served. All these so-called cheeses are nothing but chemical products that have close to nothing in common with natural cheese. (Cheese is nothing but spoiled milk. And what is milk?) All these products are made with chemicals, sodium, fat, and chemical spices to "brainwash" the taste buds.

Young children and older children as well, should snack on raw fruits and vegetables, homemade baked goods and whole foods. Babies used to get mother's milk for a year or more, and then would slowly be introduced to vegetables and fruit, all home prepared. This should be the absolute rule. Too many children are simply undernourished, not because they eat too small of portions; we have the most overfed and undernourished children in the world, right here in our country. These poor children are undernourished in spite of the formula, abundant dairy foods, Gerber baby foods and so many others. We raise our children in an era of artificial environment and nutrition yet would like them to grow up healthy? How could they?

Please do your own research on food additives, it will surprise and sicken you, but knowledge is power and it is within your power to protect your family from those who would sell their health for a few pennies profit

Did Dentists and Doctors invent our Holidays?

A fact that may not surprise you is that most home-schooling children eat much better than their neighbors who attend the public miss-education facilities. It is part of the whole philosophy of those who decided to walk that path. These kids are typically breast-fed for a much longer time and are significantly more exposed to nature. Yet, not among all of the homeschooling families, it is true. Many of the

homeschooling families are pretty overwhelmed by the stress and hard work of doing everything by themselves, that they reach out for easier solutions as well, and the junk food and malnutrition is part of it.

Baked goods are addictive as well. Not officially, but they are. It is part of the cultural standards children grow into. The biggest concern mothers have when their child's birthday is coming up is the birthday cake. Well, I wish that someday this horrible and damaging trend could be replaced by a less harmful means of birthday entertainment.

I once suggested gathering up all the children and allow them to participate in the mixing and baking of the cake, and as part of the festivities, celebrate that the cake had no poison in it. The idea went over like a lead balloon, I was considered a party wrecker and a rather odd person in general. Imagine, a mom who cared enough about her children to hope each birthday cake signified the beginning of another year of health and I was the oddball.

I would do it this way: I would gather all the fresh, natural ingredients for a delicious, healthy cake, and would allow each child who wants to participate, to have a role in the preparation process. This way the healthy cake would not be a punishment in any sense, and the idea could "grow wings", causing the children to go home and ask for the same thing on their birthdays. It may sound as though it cannot work, but it certainly can. It worked great with my own children and grandchildren.

Imagine instead of rushing to the supermarket to choose all the dreadful snacks and sugar-laden junk, standing in line for a good while - simply open your pantry knowing you have all the necessary ingredients to create a wonderful party. You would simply decide to use your time in a much wiser way. Making a cake from scratch does take more time than opening a box, that is for fact. When we invite children into our kitchens, everything takes longer to accomplish but look at the gift you are giving. Besides the obvious physically healthier children you raise, you are also giving of yourself. It takes no effort to buy a cake and not much more to buy the box mix and toss it in the oven yourself. However, involving a group of excited children into your kitchen to mix, blend and frost will create some mess, and be a little bother, but what a valuable outcome? Though you are not responsible directly for the health of your children's friends, it may surprise you one day, when after being the weird mom who doesn't buy the super-sized-sugared up birthday cakes, to discover at your front door, one of the Doubting Thomas mothers, asking for advice about her child's allergies, hyperactivity, etc.

Why is it, when we throw an adult party, we have no problem setting boundaries on what will be tolerated in our homes? No smoking, no alcohol, sugar- free, meat- free, gluten free etc. Yet, we feel pressured to join the crowd, and serve plates of poison to our precious children. Simply begin the process when your child is young, and you will never have to convince him/her otherwise. Helping your young children to understand healthy boundaries in eating, will also be a gateway to the boundaries you will need to set as the child grows, and other dangerous habits begin to look interesting.

Convert common recipes into healthy ones

Better ideas for baking for celebrations and for every day.
Replace:

White sugar -use either Stevia or fresh squeezed fruit juice, honey, organic maple syrup, ripe banana.

White flour - use instead flours such as tapioca, potato, rice, garbanzo bean, or coconut flour rice flour, Teff, buckwheat, quinoa, etc.

Vanilla can be derived directly from the vanilla bean and can be purchased organic.

Ground lemon peel adds delicious taste to many cakes and baked goods.

Instead of eggs, you can use flax seeds and chia seeds.

Baking Soda can be the healthy kind that has no aluminum.

Instead of oil, use freshly blended green apple puree. (Helps in all liver related illnesses as well as weight watch).

Instead of dairy milk, use fresh fruit juice, almond milk, sesame seeds milk, or rice milk.

Instead of chocolate use organic chocolate or avocado (when mixed with almond milk and fresh vanilla)

Giggling Dr. Green

Frosting can be made from cocoa powder mixed with almond cream or avocado to form a heavy thick cream (to thicken it further you can use Arrowroot).

Perhaps it does not look as yummy as the fancy store bought cakes with the heavy frosting; however, please remember that children learn what they live. Telling the children that processed foods are bad for them, will only help if they can eat tasty replacements. Imagine placing fresh, edible flowers on your child's birthday cake? What a sensation that would cause among the other children. Perhaps some thin shavings of ginger or berries atop the cake will make it one to remember. It is our responsibility to create a home where your children learn the joy in doing the right things. They should never feel deprived but encouraged that they are the special ones, the ones who receive nothing but the best at their table, celebration and feast. If this would be the cake we introduce, this is what they will learn is the best, just like with any other food. If you are one of those wise parents who never introduces your child to white sugar, your child will never miss it. Children cannot become addicted to something they never experience. Usually, the love for a certain food or event has grown out of positive associations. The whole fuss around birthdays is a big deal for every child and even adults. If the proper healthy food were to be introduced at these times, the child will always connect it with happiness and celebration.

Healthy food was for many years in the past associated with somewhat boring; drab, poor tasting food in many cases. Now, the awareness and care for good healthy food woke up a long line of very creative people who appreciate their lives and their families' lives as well. So, there are millions of just absolutely delicious recipes in books and available online for very healthy and very tasty foods. Just spend a bit of time looking for them.

The common birthday cake is a concoction of ingredients that should not be authorized by the FDA to be labeled as fit for human consumption and never labeled as edible or food. The birthday parties usually do not even take place in the children's homes anymore, because these little ones get so high on all the sugars that they turn into uncontrollable whirlwinds of manic energy and bounce off the walls. We take our children to places such as Chuck e cheese for their parties, where the noise level alone is enough to cause them to be over stimulated. Mix in the dairy and unlimited soda to have a recipe for disaster. I would be very interested to know how many birthday children, and their guests, do not make it home without having to vomit after such a celebration in gluttony and fool heartedness.

Giggling Dr. Green

Let us consider, for just a moment, that perhaps it would not be so terrible, if one birthday a year was the only time your child was exposed to that type of senseless eating. Well, does the child have any siblings? Surely, they will be at that party. Does the child have any friends, go to school, and attend church or synagogue? What about cousins? The list is endless, and by the time your child is in school, he could be eating "party foods" every week. Now take a look at holidays. Easter, and Valentine's Day are wonderful excuses to allow your children to jeopardize their health. I have saved the worst offender for last. Halloween is a feast for the pocketbooks of dentists and doctors. What in the world are we teaching our children on this ridiculous holiday, anyways? All year we warn them severely against even speaking to strangers, but tonight we send them out to knock on doors and ask strangers for candy? Look at that word with me please.

Candy

Allows you to

Need dentures younger

Getting back to the question; what if we allowed our children complete sugar to abandon one or two days a year? That would not be too bad right? I will let you decide. A good friend of mine called me the day after Halloween a few years ago and told me how sick her normally healthy son was. He was not vomiting nor did he have a fever or diarrhea, however, at the age of 13, he had suddenly lost the ability to control his bladder. He had wet his bed repeatedly on Halloween night and in the morning was so terribly weak. Of course - his mother was very concerned. Her description sounded like juvenile diabetes had developed overnight, so a sudden and serious attack, proved unfortunately in the emergency room to which I sent her immediately with that suspicion in mind. The large amount of candy he had consumed on Halloween had triggered juvenile diabetes. It has been a factor in his health ever since and will continue to throughout his life.

We probably feel helpless and guilty, unable to do anything about it. These celebrations have been ingrained so deeply in our culture and make us feel powerless attempting to change them. Maybe, but, we are responsible for our child's well-being. That means that we MUST draw the line and avoid our children's intoxications. We would not fail to do so when our children start to reach out for alcohol and drugs, no matter their age. However, as babies, toddlers, and young children, why don't we speak out against the "legal" drugs daily offered to our children? If your child had a peanut allergy, you would make certain this generally considered healthy food, be kept far from her/him. Thus, sugars, caffeine, food coloring, additives, preservatives, are just as or even more dangerous. Offer tasty attractive alternatives and your children will grow up naturally loving the healthiest foods possible. We must draw solid lines for our children's well-being and my friend, if you are not able to do it with a toddler, how will you be able to do it with a teenager when it will binge on alcohol and drugs?

When Omrie was still a toddler and allergic to wheat and dairy, her mother would let the party hosts know about it ahead of time. Either the host would prepare some non-dairy and gluten-free goodies for Omrie or Maayan, her mom, would prepare for Omrie her personal cake and the proper snacks to send along with her. Omrie was made to feel special; she understood how much her mother cared about her health, and never complained about not being able to eat the pretty poisons that the other children were eating. Omrie was never endangered with the foods that were toxic for the other children, even those that seemingly did not suffer from allergies. As would be expected with such a caring mother, Omrie continues to enjoy good health and celebrations mean delicious treats to her; deprivation is not in her vocabulary.

As for myself, as I am highly gluten and lactose intolerant. I love cakes and other baked goods and snacks, however I never eat any that are not good for me. I am very happy with the huge gluten and dairy free variety available and have never felt left out. There is a way we can keep our kids away from all these harmful, addictive, poisonous foods even at the biggest celebrations. Create in your children the notion that they are as precious as pure gold and as unique as a snowflake and they will grow to believe in themselves, apart from the crowd. To be different is everybody's dream. Whether to become a celebrity, or being exceptional and valuable. So, why can't we be unique in the way we chose for our children a greater appreciation for life, health, and nature?

* For more detailed research please read

"The China Study", "May All Be Fed", and "Diet for a new America"

Chapter four

Children's Playground

Israel has always been thirsty for a good rainy season as most of the year the ground is extremely dry, similar to so many other desert-like regions throughout Africa and the Middle East. What passes for a drought in America would be an improvement in Israel at times!

As I grew up in Israel right after the Second World War, to our luck the toy industry was still in its infancy. I recall the welcome times of rain as the most enjoyable and creative times of my childhood. I do not think we had much more than a ball and a few card games. All the rest was created by our own imagination; a wonderful childhood play, rich in creative discoveries. Therefore, the rainy season brought us kids buckets of fun and stimulated our rich dream world and fantasy in ways holding a beeping, blinking electronic toy never could have. The saturated soil, (since it was so dry it took a while for the water to penetrate into the soil), got so slick that it turned into an "ice skating" rink for us. Who really cared if it was really ice or just a brown muddy mess? Our parents may have cared about the mess we were not only in, but became, however they were wise enough to let us play to our heart's content for no other choice. We could not have cared less about the happy hippos we resembled and blissfully spent every daylight moment out in the glorious mud. We had invented the original "Slip and Slide" , no assembly required!

A favorite organized game during these fabulous days of mess and mayhem was a game we called "Lands." We would mark a big circle on the ground, and divide it into as many slices as the number of players we were. Imagine a giant pie, with a child standing in each slice of land. Our objective was to occupy as much land from our neighbor until he or she would literally lose their land. The only toy we had was the knife we had borrowed from the kitchen. We threw it into the soil, drew a line, yet only if we could stretch all the way to draw that line, which was our newly occupied territory. We were so deeply involved in the game and stayed at it as long as our parents would allow. The fact that we had no store bought toys forced us to use our imaginations, and create better games that have ever been sold at the giant "Toys R Us" stores. Not only were we very creative, but even more important was our constant interaction with nature and friends in all weather conditions. In front of our house was an enormous playground, and really was our only play room; the houses were so small, no one I knew had a playroom in their home, and we were happily many years away from the horrific practice of a TV in every room, let alone the computer and "Game Kid" games that have added as much to childhood disease and obesity as any junk food ever sold. We interacted with each other, played for hours together and never thought we were missing anything. The games had very strict rules and we would insist on watching and keeping these rules. Unfortunately, today many children do not interact at all, as long as they can watch TV, and play their Game Boy or any number of other electronic games, and of course, be munching on something not necessarily healthy the whole time.

We were lean, healthy children; not one of us had high blood pressure, high cholesterol, cancer or diabetes. I remember how in the hot summer days, during the long summer vacation from school, we stayed home while our father went to work. At those times, the word babysitter was not even in any household vocabulary. That was the best time to have a few of our neighborhood friends over and play our improvised games for many hours. No one ever said there is nothing to do. During those sizzling summer days when even healthy children can get lethargic and lazy, we would sit on the cool tile floor and play with just five small rocks we would find in the yard. To find rocks was easy since streets were not paved and discovering an interesting rock of just the right size and shape, well, that was a treasure worth guarding.

The ball games we played included a form of basketball and soccer and intense games, so we needed the sidewall of a house to play against. These games not only required a lot of interaction, including the occasional scuffle of course, but they were a real blessing for our basic coordination skills, our large muscle development, concentration, counting, memory, attention, creative imagination, fine motor skills, social interaction skills, self-confidence, coordination of eyes and hands, eyes and feet, focus, and overall what we all need in childhood for coordination enhancement and development. Like jumping rope for many hours, hide and seek, and stick ball (our version of baseball). Those simple games enabled us to develop all the skills we needed in order to grow up, strong and healthy with robust cardiovascular activity, with a sense of independence and well coordinated. It kept us constantly in a healthy electromagnetic environment because we were continuously in direct contact with the soil and sun outdoors. We were not exposed at any time to the damaging electromagnetic static fields that children today are regularly overly exposed to, by using cell phones, countless hours spent in front of computers and TV, video and games, tablets, too many hours indoors ,walking on synthetic fiber carpets and sitting on synthetic fiber couches.

I expect some of my dear readers to ask, "Well, this is our reality in today's culture. What can we do about it? We can't fight the way our children are influenced by their peers." Some of you may even be wondering if I am suggesting we all carve out a cozy home in the hills and live like cavemen. Honestly, I do not see the solutions as being unattainable, complicated, or drastic. I realize that those of you who live in an urban high rise may believe keeping their children well connected to nature may be difficult, but it doesn't have to be and any effort is surely a deposit into their health bank.

I do have some suggestions for you and I trust that once you begin to think about it you will come up with many more good ideas of your own.

Even in the city it is possible to take the children to the park or beach, before they tear them all down to put up more parking lots. New York City has one of the most beautiful parks in America and all across this beautiful country there are still many to be found, little areas of raw land that are available for our enjoyment, before the bulldozers and cement trucks come along and improve everything to death.

Children, with our help and encouragement, can learn to refrain from the TV and computer for at least 2-3 hours a day and do things that are connected and related to the great outdoors. We all need a regular connection with fresh air and bare earth just as every other creature on the planet does, for our physical health and emotional stability.

Children need the outdoors as plants need the sun, there really is no difference. Children who are not exposed to fresh air get sick and their development compromised. Even though they do not create chlorophyll like plants do in the sun, their bones, skin, eyes, vitamins, metabolism, and their whole vital equilibrium is dependent upon regular outdoors activity. Try to keep a plant or an animal caged indoors for a little while and witness the pitiful results, probably much sooner than you expect.

By being connected to mother earth's vital energy, children can learn to grow their own vegetables. Even a small flower pot on a sunny balcony or even the windowsill can help foster a sense of nature in a city child. We can introduce our kids to soil and nature, even under less than ideal conditions. Find ways to draw your child's attention to the seasonal changes. Not only through movies and

TV, please. We can initiate crafts during which our children collect fall leaves and create a beautiful piece of art. Take your child on a nature walk, even in the city. Help your child to create a journal, noting the types of birds, trees, flowers and insects you both encounter. Please do not discourage the child who finds joy in the lowly pigeon, or hurry along the youngster who stops to watch ant toil with a heavy crumb. These are just the types of early experiences that help our children grow to be compassionate individuals, who are healthy in body, mind and spirit.

Take your child to the farmer's market, to purchase the freshest local foods available. Encourage his help in selecting the produce, and if he occasionally chooses something you would not, all the better, you are both learning and growing each day. Children are so often our best teachers; no one has had time to tell them not to be excited at each new day, and if they are lucky, no one ever will.

When you get home from the market, allow your little buddies to help you wash and prepare the luscious foods you have brought home. You may wish to get in the habit of purchasing a bit more than your meal will require, for eating on the way home, and during preparation will get you less of the final planned dish. I suggest no limit on the amount of fresh foods you make available to your child. If you keep clean, cut vegetables in the fridge, in a bowl right at the front that is what your child will reach for. The same is true for a bowl of fruit on the table, so pretty, no other table decoration is necessary and so healthy. Imagine if every doughnut in America was instantly replaced with a piece of fruit! That one miracle would induce such an increase in overall health in the nation; the MEGA Force may begin to quiver in fear.

Are you concerned your child will cut her/his little fingers helping with the salad making? The very youngest child can be shown how to tear the greens, snap the ends off beans and pull each little silk from the fresh corn, As the child grows a bit, and you teach her/him how to use the knife, she/he may have a slip or two, but they will learn and their pride will be priceless. Those wonderful little hands should learn the coordination it requires to prepare food, all the while enjoying the delicate smells of the fresh vegetables separate, and then in combination. Make kitchen work a game for your children and each meal will present another joyful opportunity to prepare them for their own game of life one day, getting closer to you and them and having the best memories for life. There are no real life experiences to be found in front of the TV or the popular "Play like a Zombie Station". Real life does not consist of killing cops, stealing cars, and selling drugs, which makes up the script for some of today's most popular video games. Real life is not just changing TV channels with a remote, while eating super-sized portions of foods that are only good for supersizing ourselves. The chemically engineered junk foods our children become addicted to are specially formulated to destroy their taste buds. To receive the same enjoyment from eating, they constantly require more sugar and salt, just like a drug addict who is always looking for a new and more powerful way to devastate themselves. Junk foods are certainly a part of the reason why the teen escapes to drugs, there is nothing left to experience, and life has no value, as proved in the violent video games.

Imagine yourself having to run your adult life, with all its responsibilities such as preparing your own food, managing your budget, making wise purchases, choosing friends with caution, even launder clothes and complete an employment application, without any preparations. We ask the same of our children when we allow them to waste away their childhood and youth as well as their very health, on mindless activities that require little or no physical movement or mental effort. That screen which gets bigger with each passing year, as though it is vital that we allow it to dominate our homes, creates the biggest problems for today's youth that occasionally I wish it had never been invented. Of course, there are worthy programs, but even during those what are the commercials about? McDonald's, Jack-that is less nutritious than the-Box it comes in, or how about the house of roasted cows, Arby's. Directly after the commercials you either run to the drive through and buy fast food, or order to have food delivered, if getting in your car seems like an ordeal. Next are the advertisements for all the wonderful quick cures for all the wonderful food you were just encouraged to buy. Personally, I do not understand why stomach ache medicine is not a condiment, so we can ask for it on our burger bun, rather than have to bother purchasing it separately. Don't be afraid, even as I write this, there is probably someone considering marketing an idea similar to that ridiculous one. Children are force fed with information they need never know, such as "How to manage your life with a drug for every problem". How sad is that? Our children must have time to initiate, create, overcome obstacles, enjoy success and achievements, live through failure, get up, and try again.

Do our children know how to gather firewood, make an emergency shelter, which plants are safe and edible, or even how to wash clothes without electricity if necessary? Children quite naturally enjoy adventure, so create opportunities for them to be successful under unusual conditions. Scouting is one of the best-organized activities still popular in America. If you do not have a troop in your area, or choose not to involve your child in scouting for whatever reason, please, do supply your child with similar lessons and experiences that participating in scouting would. For those of you who do encourage your child's wilderness spirit, you will find indescribable pleasure on your child's face as you allow imaginative play. From Robinson Crusoe, to the Swiss Family Robinson, there are so many wonderful stories you can share with your children that will inspire their play.

Our children have the right and need to prepare themselves not just for an adult life, but also for basic survival. We live in uncertain times and as parents must, without alarming our children, help them to be able to care for themselves in an emergency. This can happen easily if you make a game out of it. Play math games, cooking games, laundry and chore games. Ask your children a lot of "what if" questions so you can determine what they are thinking and where their fears are. Stretch your child's ability to climb, crawl, run and jump. Teach them to make a fishing pole and find bait, how to pitch a tent and what the different clouds mean. Does your child know to follow water downhill if ever lost in a mountain? Does she/he realize that petting a cute bear cub could bring a raging momma bear running at them? Do your children know how to tell how deep the water is in a river? There are tremendous resources available to guide you in your child's survival education, and if you are at all like me you will enjoy the task immensely.

To contribute to the changes our children have to undergo in order to be able to face reality, and yet enjoy life with all its challenges can be a fun task and quality time together well spent. These are all skills that can be learned in a playful and enjoyable way, and if the "Toys R Us" stores are not willing to market simple toys geared towards your child's development, create your own. A hammer, some wood, and a jar of nails will amuse a child for hours. Your children need to know how to sew, make a rag rug, and cook. By the way, although there are traditional roles, I believe in boys and girls knowing how to do everything and having opportunities to practice their skills. Eventually their own natural desires will surface, however they will have had the experiences to draw on should they ever need them. The "Toys R Us" stores must always be marketing something new that is louder and requires more batteries than last year's model or their profit will drop. Toy stores do sell wood blocks, crayons, jump ropes and balls of every size and color, but they sure do not make much room for them. I suggest making your child's toys yourself and when they grow up a little, with them. As I write this, there is a terrible controversy over toys from China having lead paint in them. China has also sent poisonous toothpaste to America along with some pet food that was lethal as well. Again; read the labels, know where the products you are buying are made and if there is something you do not understand on a label, remember - it is always safe to wait. Do not buy today what may be recalled tomorrow. The more we stick to nature's offerings, the safer we are.

Johnny's room was a Toy Store

When Johnny was sick and I was called to treat him his room looked like a toy store. He was bathed in so many toys it seemed as though he would be buried under them. As I glanced around the room I wondered when he had time for creativity. Where can his imagination run wild?

The molded plastic of every color crowded his room forced this little boy to live with a constant flow of heavy electrostatic fields surrounding him. When I commented my thoughts to his mother she said; "Oh really? I guess I just never thought about it that way." It was too much, too crowded, too stimulating, too polluting the air in his room, and simply put; unhealthy for an 18 months old baby.

I am not surprised why so many children need special education classes, Ritalin medications and counseling for their so-called attention deficit disorders. The hyperactive- child has not been allowed to play and exercise his large muscles outdoors enough. Keeping children cooped up indoors in front of electronic equipment is like shifting a car into fifth gear, and accelerating while holding the hand brake at the same time. Children must utilize their energy and experience the fantastic feeling of achievements. The child must be allowed to regularly enjoy the feeling of creativity, and of getting results for their efforts. Children who do not get these needs met are unhealthy, unhappy and restless and the cost of their toys will not save them. The complete healthy development of their hopes and dreams will not function appropriately and the child will start to display signs of a wild animal in captivity. Refuse Mozart's piano, do not allow Edison to experiment, and tell Marie Curie that 4-year-old little girls do not need to know how to read. What is electronically hypnotized child learning? These are additional real reasons for ADD, ADHD, learning disabilities etc. When they will no longer sit quietly in front of their electronic babysitters then they must be medicated. The child who asks too many questions in class will not be tolerated. The youth who looks out the window to watch a bird build a nest is rebuked. After the Ritalin and its ugly cousins have been in use a while more diseases begin to pop up, such as bipolar disorders, schizophrenia, depression, obesity, anorexia, anxiety, cancer, and arthritis, just to name a few. Can you imagine how it could have been had your child had the choice of actively playing outdoors, on a regular basis? How much healthier could the child be if only he had been guided and exposed to "hard work" by building the tallest Lego tower ever or planting his own little yard, or, building her own dollhouse with her mom and dad?

Giggling Dr. Green

The reasons for the very unhealthy generation growing up today are many. Nevertheless, there is so much light at the end of the tunnel as we are not doomed to raise sickly children; we can choose to be proactive and change their living conditions. Children are so delicate and raising them must be done with one hundred percent of our commitment and creative thinking. No childcare, no nanny and no babysitter, electronics can replace our natural instincts and senses of what is the best for our child. Please think about it. Please go back to your inner child and ask yourself the question, "Would I rather play with my mom and daddy, or have a big house and a big new car, yet not have my dear parents to play with? Would I rather sit in front of the TV and eat junk or play outdoors barefooted in the sand?"

Please reach inside your heart, find your innocent feelings, be honest with yourself. It is the little child in yourself who can help you heal yourself and the little child you raise? This is the Giggling Dr. Green who is talking to you. Allow your child to giggle together with you.

Choosing games for our children must not be considered a mundane task. It must be done through the scrutinizing eye of a loving parent with a vision and a dream for that child's future. Envision our child growing up, turning into a happy, successful, and healthy adult. Let us keep in mind that every game and every toy contributes to our child's development. Won't we choose only the best influence for our children? It is absolutely up to our input, judgment and intelligent choices, how our children will thrive. Moreover, this is what we really would like to see our children do - thrive. Healthy, happy and well taken care of children grow to be adults who will positively influence the future of our and their world. The next generation can be what we really would like it to be. Not like these elderly ladies shaking their heads saying; "The kids today are awful". I strongly disagree. They are good children; they just need to be protected from the different industries that have just one vision – their own bank accounts. I think we need to apologize to our children for these greedy manufacturers that forgot they were kids, and God only knows - maybe suffer from sad and unhappy children of their own. Could it possibly be Karma? Let us change it and make a difference.

Chapter five
Crime rates in schools are soaring

Turning on the nightly news has become a practice in morbidity. Take for example the cruelty, the crime, and unspeakable horror stories we learn about from the reporters, the victims, and sometimes even the criminals themselves. How far has human deprivation gone that even children are now committing many of the most horrendous crimes and often against each other. It is very hard to consider this but as parents we must look into our home life when a child goes so terribly off course. What has the child been watching on TV? Which movies were they allowed to view? And what types of games did they play? We cannot surround our children with bubble wrap as much as we may like to, however, we can control what happens in our homes and we can provide our children with a solid foundation of personal responsibility and values. The games of death and destruction our children play do not show the grieving families, the shattered dreams or the years of torment even a survivor of a horrible crime goes through. Who has forgotten the tragedy at Columbine School in Colorado and more recently at Virginia Tech University, where a young man who had earlier been deemed mentally ill shot 32 students and faculty members to death? It is rather poignant to mention here that one of the teachers killed that day was a wonderful man who had survived the Holocaust. Imagine that he had survived the hate machine that was Nazi Germany but was shot to death by a troubled youngster here in America. The young man concluded his reign of terror by killing himself, and so, once again, a tragedy ends with no one to stand accountable for the horror.

What do your children do when they come home from school? Is schoolwork before TV? Or a little healthy snack at the kitchen table with you to talk over their day? Do your children have responsibilities? Or maybe a pet to care for? I would not only limit TV time, but also hide the remote. At least require them to cross the huge gaping living room to change the channel! You must realize that the ideas thrust upon our children come with no accountability, and the children are too young to determine for themselves what is right or wrong in all these abstract situations. Liviu Librescu, the fine professor from Romania I honored in the last paragraph, understood hate; he had looked it in the eye once before and lived to tell about it. This time, when he saw it coming towards his students he decided their young lives, 20 of them, were worth more than his own.

Giggling Dr. Green

He stood and held the door telling his students to flee and taking five bullets before he fell dead. Will your child grow up to make a choice like that someday? We hope, of course, that that day will never come, but if it does, will he be the shooter, or the hero? The choices begin at home. At 63 years old, my beloved husband can still be brought to tears by a sad part in even a cartoon. Where is the compassion in today's youth? Who will be the heroes of tomorrow?

Can you remember a movie that touched you so deeply that not only did you dwell on it for days, but years after seeing it, it still brings memories of pain, sadness, fear, or better yet, hope and encouragement? "Remember the Titans" is one of those movies for me. I watch it every once in a while to remind myself that there have always been those people who will stand for what is right about America and fight to change that which is wrong. If you do not stand for something, you will fall for anything. As adults, we all have movies that bring certain emotions to the surface and we see ourselves as mature, understanding what ethical behavior is and must be. But our children, they are much more impressionable than we are and therefore fantasy and fact are not so easily discerned. If we parents do not stand firm on what "entertainment" we allow our children to participate in, who will? Will we blame the English professor, who saw the troubled youth disturbed writings, yet did not report them? Will we blame the University for not issuing a more thorough warning sooner? Or will we finally stand up and say; I will raise my child to know right from wrong and it is my responsibility to monitor what he does, and who he is spending his time with. In a day when a 10 year old has to stand in front of a judge for murder or a 12 year old is in a detention center for raping a 3 year old, how can we close our eyes to the influences of the world? I am almost sure that these children are not pathological criminals. I want to believe that these kids are just under the influence of an industry of TV, movies and video-games that teach no self-control, and offer no consequences for bad choices. A TV in your child's bedroom is an open door to disaster. Not only will they watch too much for their own physical health, but their moral compass will become shattered in a reckless blur of right and wrong. Is the TV your child's babysitter? Then I must be bold, and tell you to change your priorities quickly.

Children who have a pet to care for typically grow to value life. A child that understands the responsibility of helping the family vegetable garden to grow will generally not be the one aiming a gun at his own mother. The child, who takes fresh food to a lonely neighbor, will not be among those who are caught throwing rocks at her windows.

Giggling Dr. Green

In his book Dr. Clarkson tells how he grew up in a single parent family. His mother was very poor and worked hard just to feed her children. Even with her difficult life, she had rules for them to follow and one of the unbreakable ones was that each child must spend at least 2 hours a day reading. Even though as a child, Dr. Clarkson had been diagnosed with learning difficulties, through his mother's diligence and encouragement, he grew to be renowned for his knowledge, skills and values.

So, please do not try to protest that you are too busy to enforce reasonable rules in your home. If you are honestly unable to control what your children watch on TV, get rid of it! The same goes for video games, and computer games. We have to face reality, assume responsibility and decide how we would like to shape our kids' future; therefore the world they will live in. Do we want to live in a world run by crime just because we could not find the time to supervise our children's entertainment?

When watching unmonitored TV, our children also get many lessons in how to pop a pill to cure any problem, be it a physical, mental or sexual discomfort. Children must be guided to understand the correct and positive influences for their future skills dealing in the world of adulthood, responsibility and independence. We are obligated to support and guide them. For the future of our children, the new car, the payment of the new TV, and the mortgage payments are irrelevant. Children have grown up many generations without a plasma TV, in smaller houses and with one, less expensive car. Yet, they grew up at home and with a parent always nearby. We must examine our own priorities. Once we decide to have a child, she/he must be the top priority, regardless of budget, titles or career promotions. Our children have sadly been demoted to the lowest place on the priority list. We find the cheapest babysitter or childcare center; we find "good TV programs" ; we have all the "support" to raise our kids from others, and with as many modern tools as possible. Remember how children would crawl on the floor and mom and dad would just spend time playing with them? This must be our normal, daily scenario. If you feel that you must reach all the other material, career or status goals, better think twice before you have a child. Every child must be the number one on our priority list. It will not be solved with money, a new SUV or a room full of plastic, battery operated, no imagination required toys. The kids need more than anything else, the loving mother's touch, every evening when they go to bed and whenever they hurt or are scared. Daddy has to be present every evening at the dinner table and be available to his children. "How was school?" and "Did you finish your homework?" is the extent of conversation many parents have with their children and it is clearly not sufficient.

Giggling Dr. Green

Playing with your children is educating them with the skills and values we really would like them to have. We can't expect them to learn from watching movies and playing video games; quite the opposite When they are teenagers and we start pulling our hair, unable to understand how yesterday 's sweet baby became today's anti-social, non-communicative ball of anger; we will have to admit we allowed it to happen.

Protect children from the harmful media

I really do not want any one of you to think that I would try to get us back to the Stone Age. I would never say that there are no worthwhile, caring medical doctors, and I do recognize there are times, particularly in an emergency, when surgery and prescription medication are necessary. Do you suppose for a severed limb I would not rush a loved one to the hospital? Of course I would. There is a time and a place for everything of value and when things are used in moderation and wisdom, great good can be derived from many sources.

Computers, electronics and all types of media fall into the same category. It is necessary for many parts of our child's development in the learning process. It is also very important in our day and age for our children to be well equipped to work in the technology fields of tomorrow. The problem, as in many things, is the balance between the child's needs for their education and development and their needs for good physical health. The health needs must be at the very top spot on the priority list. The time frame for children to experience different types of media has to be in accordance with their age and current condition.

When Jim returns home from daycare, he cannot wait; he just has to watch, just as so many children do, for the 200th time, his favorite program. It is important to him; yet, his mom should make sure that he does not spend more than just a daily maximum of 30 minutes in front of the screen. He is just 2 years old, and with all the respect to the peace and quiet we like at home, a damaging situation for the child should be the vital consideration.

His older siblings are already addicted to soap operas and spend a few hours each day in front of the TV, anxious to see who will do what to whom, next. Wouldn't you agree that there is absolutely no educational or developmental benefit in watching soap operas? Lea would have the best babysitter in the world watching TV since she was a baby and so did her brother, Ross. The children get so many distorted messages from those cheap TV programs, their values are seriously compromised.

Giggling Dr. Green

The ways soap opera characters solve relationship problems is clearly not a good model for anyone to learn by and use for a happy, healthy, honest and committed future relationship. Why wouldn't a parent set rules and boundaries to these types of exposures? Why can't responsible parents guide their children to truthful values and creative activities? Because they either do not know any better, or, because the time they need to invest in changing their children's path in their growing process, is too consumed by different, "more important" issues. Even by taking a nap instead of being with the children. Chatting with a friend instead of reading with your children or playing with them, or initiating other constructive activities.

Playing with our children should not be a chore, or a task. Playing with our children is, in my understanding, the most important part in their healthy, happy, and creative upbringing. It is even more important than a gourmet meal or a shiny clean home; I truly think so.

When we lived in the South of the Dead Sea in Israel, I had a house full of children. My husband's two young boys from his first marriage and my daughter from my first marriage gave us three children in the same age group. Then, we had two more boys together, and, for a whole year, I had my niece due to a tragedy in my sister's life. When they all were still very young, I would spend the whole day with them. We would ride bikes together, go for runs, walks, swimming, ball games, and play tennis. When the weather had us stay indoors, we would do a lot of art and crafts. The house was one hundred percent a children's paradise. I never felt it to be my duty or in any way a burden. I saw it as a wonderful opportunity to reclaim my own child and act upon it. We had a lot of fun together and the children learned everything I would like them to by doing everything together. Not by a babysitter who could not educate them by the same belief system, the values, tastes, ideas, energy and love, I could give them naturally. They did not need the long hours of TV. They were not overweight, and had no eating disorders. They would go to sleep at 8:30 PM and then my husband and I had the rest of the evening to ourselves, to do whatever we would like or need to do. When I was a single, divorced mom, I certainly had my share of men who wanted to date me; however, since Maayan was the most important person in my life, and she was 1 year old, I would never leave her with my mother or babysitter to accept any invitation. The quality time with my daughter was sacred. It was my commitment to her before she was born. That I am hers and she was mine, and nothing and no one would be more important than our togetherness. With the other children, later on in my life, I had the very same agreement. Today, I celebrate children who have no drug issues, no violence issues, no alcohol and our relationships are just way beyond my very sweetest dreams. Their values are so much higher than mine ever were at their age. Their devotion to their children is so wonderful, that I said to my daughter, "In my dreams, I would have wished you could have been my mother, I am so proud of you and envy the children, for you are such a wonderful mother".

However, Maayan spent her early childhood away from the TV. In those days, there was no computer and cell phones were only in Jules Verne's vast imagination. In 1863, Jules Verne wrote a novel about a young man who lived in a world of glass skyscrapers, high-speed trains, gas-powered automobiles, calculators, and a worldwide communications network, yet amidst all the wondrous inventions and improvement, he is miserable. The novel, "Paris in the 20th Century" could easily be written today and be autobiographical about countless individuals who trade families for a bigger house or newer car.

The hours children spend in front of the TV do not only rob them of their healthy belief system and introduce them to many very unfortunate truths about the adult world, it also robs them of the ability and right to develop a healthy, creative, and naturally innocent world of imagination. As I already mentioned before, I do not think there is anything better and healthier in our mental, emotional, physical and spiritual balance and health than a well-developed innocent and clear imagination. Children must all be encouraged to enjoy and act out wonderful fantasies such as the "Wizard of Oz", Robinson Crusoe, or Captain Hook. The TV robs our children of their naivety and creates very unhealthy, disturbed values and sick concepts about life. Please, be aware of it since electronic media is a vital part in every household today. I recall this horrifying time when I was in Israel, when the suicide bombers were just part of the daily routine, almost in every living room the entire day into the night - on TV. I felt that in such times, when my grandchildren are basically in the front line and are exposed to this direct anti-children war, it is time for me to be there with them. I broke down; I could not take the vivid TV reports that left nothing to the imagination. Young children would be with their parents watching the ugliest and most horrifying visions of humankind. Do we grasp what these poor little children have to deal with in their young imaginations? How has their beautiful world of rainbows and butterflies been replaced by blood, death, fear, grief and terror?

Yes, I completely broke down and could not watch it with my family. I suggested keeping the children busy, making jewelry and painting with them instead of watching TV. The same goes for all the news in every part of the world. Just like the embryo in the womb needs separation and protection from the outer world, so do children have the same need for their proper development to be protected from the sad, ugly parts of the world. Why should a 4-year-old child in America be exposed to the pictures of killed children in Iraq? The children will grow up, and in time will be stronger to deal with the unkind parts of reality. I don't suggest sugarcoating their world, yet there is no need to hurry and expose them to all this at early childhood. The time will come when they must know and face the reality of humankind's sad parts - when their understanding and comprehension matures.

At the time when suicide bombers in Israel were still a daily reality, you would hear children in the street playing "Suicide Bomber and victims". Imagine, a small child pretending to be a suicide bomber. I overheard a 3 year old tell his friends, "Hey, I didn't explode yet" Later I heard, "Do you see that car over there? That is the one I blew up inside, and all of those rocks piled up are the people I killed." These were their games. Children have to act out their fears, imaginations and perceptions, but it is our responsibility to monitor what they are exposed to. Children can learn about world events, in a language and level of information they can accept, through conversation and stories. As sad as the stories will still be, they are still not as vivid as the TV repeatedly displaying all the horror. Please be aware of the damaging effects of those horrific images. There is a reason for the crime rates climbing throughout our schools, and even in homes. Children must play and act out their impressions in order to deal with their thoughts, fears and sense of helplessness. They fear terribly not being able to protect themselves. They have to play; it is natural and beneficial; however, we have to provide them constructive and positive imagination subjects to play with instead of the destructive subjects that can lead to the most devastating disasters and tragedies.

Electronics in Children Bedrooms

My long-term experience with children's health and well-being taught me the importance of exposing children to a healthy, pure, tranquil, peaceful and unpolluted environment. Today as we all understand the concept of "good energy" and "bad energy" we understand the important role of; quality of life and the conditions required for our health.

Everything in the world has an electromagnetic field. The rocks, the water, the animals, the furniture and the flowers are all composed of electromagnetic activity. Everything in nature has an electromagnetic field. We are living beings, or, even better put, living creatures with our own unique electromagnetic field which puts us in the kingdom of nature. Well, this is a huge responsibility that we should honor as we care for our families well being. Disrupting the electromagnetic field of any element on earth, forces the creation of something different from what was intended. If, for example, a rock's electromagnetic field were to be exposed to a different electromagnetic field other than it's natural one, the rock would begin to turn into a different material. (Like glass made of sand) Our children, as all living creatures, require the proper electromagnetic field. Like the plants, wild animals, birds and the trees. We need the electromagnetic field that allows our healthy cells to function properly. From the smallest flower to the mighty elephant, we all share the same need for this proper balance for our healthy cells. In our civilization, many of these very natural, healthy electromagnetic field-balancing elements have been removed and replaced by overwhelmingly unnatural, unhealthy and harmful elements. Under the banner of better living, advanced civilization, modern life, or urban life, we have lost our well-balanced electromagnetic field and have been exposed to very disruptive and harmful electromagnetic fields. This crime against creation is no secret and I have not in any way invented or exaggerated that danger. The synthetic carpets, plastic furniture, the plastic bottles and dishes, the plastic restaurant chains indoor playgrounds, (a bonus after the mind numbing food they just ate there).The plastic inflated jump houses parents rent for their child's birthday party, the stuffed animals, the plastic backpacks, plastic shoes, even plastic clothes, cell phones, digital watches, etc, etc. All these create harmful electromagnetic field disturbances that our children are constantly being exposed to and they have no-built in defense.

This onslaught of modern living creates a constant disruption of the natural healthy cells electromagnetic field and disables the cells normal vital activity and depletes the immune system as well as the neuron transmitted vital functions. It is a source for many health problems that will later be labeled by doctors in a huge variety of different names. All that is really needed is a re-alignment of the electromagnetic field of the healthy cells, enabling them to resume their proper functioning of the self-healing mechanism, as well as the immune system by allowing an electronic media free, sleeping environment in your child's bedroom.

The ancient Chinese already knew 5000 years ago how important energy flow was and would send their patients to relax, walk or simply lay between heaven and earth every day for at least 20 minutes to an hour. Staying indoors and watching TV or being glued to the computer screen will begin the damage. All we need is to keep the bedrooms, ours as well as our children's clear of any electromagnetic polluting devices, at least throughout the restful sleeping hours.

The major furniture companies are very successful in designing tempting pieces for our children's rooms. The parents, along with the children, find the

Giggling Dr. Green

colorful, easy to clean desks, toy boxes, and even beds made of plastic or compressed laminated wood to be very appealing. There are even plastic and laminated TV stands that hold every manner of electronic component, including the video game systems. These are, I must say, deadly from the electromagnetic-field balance point of view for our children (and us as well). Ours and our children's health are not the designer's responsibility but ours. Parents, it is our responsibility to protect our children.

Try, just for an experiment, to grow a plant in a room that has a TV and a computer in it. Allow a pet, say a hamster, to have its environment up on the child's computer desk, and watch how long, and well, the little fellow can live in such a highly charged electromagnetic area. How short his life span would be and how damaged their health would be after not too long. I read an article about a man who set about proving how damaging the electromagnetic field of the cell phone is for us, and, of course our children as well. He took a raw egg, and centered it between two cell phones that called each other. The cell phones stayed connected to each other this way for an hour. The result was – a hardboiled egg. This is how powerful the cell phones are, yet, this is basically how harmful the disturbing electromagnetic field of the electronic devices are for our children. Especially in their bedrooms, which should be kept as calm, and natural as possible; a child's personal sanctuary, if you will. That plastic or laminated desk with all its electronic devices on it, should not be used by the child, and certainly not be placed in her/his room, where the very air she/he breathes as they sleep becomes polluted by positive electromagnetic charge. (As you know, we need the negative electromagnetic charge).

Children should sleep in a room made of natural elements with the lowest possible electromagnetic static field. For example; instead of any synthetic carpets, please choose organic linen or cotton rugs, tiles or wooden flooring. It is so funny when people wipe the floor and complain about the huge amounts of sand on the floor and call it a dirty floor. They simply do not realize how much better the sand on the floor is for the child than the synthetic carpet or laminate wooden floors. The beds should be made of wood, and the bed linens should be made of linen, or pure organic cotton. The lamps should be made of salt rocks or wood and covered with any natural materials; definitely not plastic. The child's sleeping clothes should be made of organic cotton, or linen; never any synthetic fibers. The cups from which your child drinks the water, shouldn't be made of plastic either of a natural product, like glass, wood or even paper or iron would serve well. Yes, even the glass we drink our water from has an electromagnetic field that interacts with our own bio-electromagnetic field we prefer to tune in together smoothly and constructively for our balance. If you can, I would highly recommend taking out all of the stuffed animals from your child's room, plastic toys should not be in the child's room and neither should all the electronics. The room your child spends the entire night, where the body recuperates and breathes to renew the energy and blood production, should be as natural as possible. When you shake the stuffed animals, or when you dust the plastic surfaced desk in your child's room, see how much dust has accumulated. If you try it in the darkness, you can see the sparks of electrostatics like the lightning.

This dust is due to the electrostatic force the plastic creates. That means that the air is polluted from the dust particles in the air that are magnetized by the static electromagnetic field of the stuffed animals or the desk. That means that the child sleeps and breathes the polluted air filled with these particles, due to the static loaded air; it prevents the clean breathing your child needs for a healthy, revitalizing sleep. Understandably the invention of the synthetic materials eased the burden of stain removal, the hassle with broken glass when children are a little clumsy and lowered the expenses. But a healthy child is the best investment ever as this saves us days missed from work, agony and worries as well as time and effort we need to spend if having to run from one doctor's appointment to the next, sleepless nights, and the pain of watching our child suffer versus the pleasure and stress-free life of living with a healthy child.

Imagine an elephant living in a synthetic environment, day and night, living off synthetic dishes, bombarded by electronics and plastic lava lamps, eating artificial junk food. Imagine how long this elephant would be able to function normally and naturally? Even an elephant would soon become sick and would probably display all the typical symptoms of restlessness, anxiety, constipation, eating disorders and sleeping disorders. The blood work would be alarming and the conditions would need to be changed immediately. (Hmm… would you like to be around the elephant when it is not constipated anymore?)

When thinking responsibly about our children's well-being and balanced health, we must help them maintain their natural needs met. These needs are not made of plastic and brass, but as close to nature as possible, even as if they were in their own little cocoon. So, it is not just the media that has this damaging electromagnetic influence on our children as well as on us , but, it is everything the modern industry developed to artificially furnish and decorate our child's environment.

However, when we go back to the media, we must consider cell phones as well, Ipods, the quick microwave dinners, the many hours children spend in the

Giggling Dr. Green

synthetic furnished rooms and so much more. In order to help them maintain good health awareness of all these little yet significant influences on our children's daily healthy balance - is required.

Himalayan Salt lamps

A crystal salt lamp in the room helps to create negative ions and improve the electromagnetic field balance in the room. The benefits of these naturally beautiful lamps are immense. While most ionizers on the market are just another man-made machine, the salt crystal lamp is a beautiful alternative of mother - nature without any noise and no harmful ozone added to our homes. Salt crystal lamps are highly beneficial for daily use in the whole house. Bedrooms, living and dining rooms and mainly near the TV and computers, to neutralize and clean the air. Use these lovely lamps to reduce your own fatigue. A crystal salt lamp near your child's computer will minimize the ill effect of the radiation and bring a soothing effect to your child's surrounding work area; they improve concentration and refresh the child naturally by neutralizing the effects of an artificial environment.

Please place a small crystal salt light in your child's room as a night light. Those lamps enrich the air with negative ions, not an electric air purifier would do. I recommend the gorgeous crystal salt lamps from the Himalayas, because the salt is mined by hand.

You will be delighted with the improved sleep and health your child will enjoy after using the salt lamps for a period of time and will want one in every room soon!

TV harms the eyes and spine

When watching TV after Bobbi returns from daycare, he lays on the couch, as the TV screen is to his right. The couch stands perpendicular to the TV. Can you see how he would lay with his head turned to the right side for an extended length of time? This is a very unnatural way of holding the head for any period of time and therefore creates a lot of tension in the neck muscles. Do you think the doctor who examines Bobbi when his throat hurts will consider his neck muscles? Well, of course not. The first stop would be checking the tonsils and recommending an antibiotic medicine. Why would he think about the connection between neck and tonsils? On the other hand, even worse, why would he think that Bobbi is spending a few hours a day laying in a crooked position on the couch fascinated by the TV? Because this is the mainstream training. When the throat is a little red, it means there is an infection in the throat, period, and end of sentence.

Giggling Dr. Green

This is not the way complementary medicine or, if you prefer, alternative medicine sees it. Why do I take the time to stress this to you? Because I would like to help you understand how your children can get sick, without getting too anxious and worried, even if the doctors think differently. I know how many of you readers, raise your brows a bit as you read this. However, if you stick with me just a little longer, you will be able to conclude whether it makes sense to you or not, and maybe, it would be better for your child to get a simple harmless chiropractic adjustment rather than a medication for the throat. The tonsillitis will recur, the medications will be reapplied and get even stronger and then the real damage will begin from the unnecessary medications' side effects and their treatments.

Imagine how the muscles function; the muscle action is by pulling, they do not push. When the muscles pull, they require certain biochemical processes which in turn produce the by-product as one of them is the lactic acid. When the muscles work the regular cycle and rhythm, like when we walk at home from one point to the next, the coordination between the muscles contraction, the muscle relaxation, the blood circulation and our breathing, will leave almost no noticeable lactic acid. So, in our daily routine we don't get the sore muscles we tend to feel after we work out, or walk an unusually long distance or through meadows we were not used to. This lactic acid is constantly broken down by the oxygen we breathe and the coordinated blood circulation to the muscles. The reason we would get the sore muscles, or muscle ache we know so well from sudden unusual muscle effort, is because the muscle did not receive sufficient oxygen while acting, and the lactic acid was not neutralized sufficiently yet. It will be, when the muscle will continue to work and contract, with much less effort yet with deep breathing. Would you think that a sore muscle after a good workout calls for antibiotics?

Now, think about Bobbi's small, tender and very young neck. He lies on the couch with his head turned for a long time to watch the TV screen. He has been so fascinated that he does not move. Just lays there for, at times an hour or maybe even longer, and watches the TV. These muscles had been contracted for a whole hour without letting up the tension even for one minute. Is this a natural position of the neck of a 3-year-old child? Certainly not.

Therefore, after a day or two, the muscles are in the process of recovering and breaking the lactic acid down, taken to the doctor. The throat will be red, because, remember, there was a distended period of time of which these muscles were poorly circulated. Are you aware of the fact that muscle ache may even be accompanied with a fever? When the lactic acid is staying for a longer period of time in the muscles, it feels and acts like an inflammation. Nevertheless, a little massage, chiropractic adjustment, a warm bath, PEMF, Reflexology, or any other means of muscle relaxation, circulation enhancement – will be the best answer. Lots of water, maybe a little herbal tea, light touch therapy, even laughter, can all work naturally together towards Bobbi's healing. There is absolutely no need for medications. This is only one little example of how children, and adults as well, can find health much faster, and many times more efficiently, before reaching out for the harmful medication. I do not try to simplify every disease, yet, I do think based upon my experience, that there are still many different ways to look and check the reasons for the child's complaints before rushing to the pharmacy aisle. Here, the media definitely played the role of harming Bobbi. It plays many more harmful roles, which I am about to elaborate upon.

The spine - Damaged from electronic screens

When children are slumped into the couch or a recliner in front of the TV, their spine, that is in its most vulnerable development stages, is severely compromised. Imagine the spine as a long chain of pearls that are just connected by a thread. When you pull this chain in any direction, it will move. Now, imagine how this pearl chain is supported by ribbons that are tied on both ends. These ribbons, when they are tight, can hold this chain straight, yet, when you let go of one of them the chain will collapse to one side.

If you decide to keep the chain straight, you had better keep the ribbons evenly long and strong.

The same way you can imagine the spine. The spine is made of the collection of vertebras that do not hold themselves upright by themselves. The vertebrae are dependent upon the muscles strength and length. When children are in their development stage, the health of their back, spine and vertebra is absolutely dependent upon the movements, activities, and balanced resting state of the child. In other words, children should sit and lay on structured surfaces and not on soft beds and soft couches. They should be encouraged to sit straight from very early on. I personally do not like to see how very young children sit in their umbrella style strollers with absolutely no support for their back. It is true that muscles do not get stronger through support. Muscles strengthen only through activity and healthy nutrition. However, when muscles are in the state of rest, they must be evenly supported in order to maintain their balance and even length. When sitting on a soft couch, the pelvis, which is at the bottom, is placed unevenly on the surface. The back will try to compensate in order to stay up right which will force one muscle group to work harder than the other muscle group. It may and usually does create back pain. In adults the back pain can be relieved by an adjustment, if this is the reason. However, children grow into bad posture habits and start to develop all the problems of scoliosis including- hyper-lordosis, which is a condition of excessive curvature in the lumbar portion of the spine, giving the child a swayback appearance, and hyper-kyphosis, which is seen in the increase of the upper spinal curves, can cause:

Hunchback, scoliosis, kiphosys, lordosys and even loss of voice or epileptic symptoms

When the back grows unhealthy and too weak to properly support the trunk, or the muscles develop too weak to hold the front part of the body, many different physical and even emotional disorders could develop. For example: Too loose belly muscles can cause constipation, gas, indigestion, bladder infections, shallow breathing, asthma symptoms, anxiety and nightmares. Imagine all these and many more issues can develop into serious health problems, just from sitting inappropriately in front of the TV without parental supervision, guidance and correction. Actually, even skin problems can start from poor TV watching habits.

We must always be mindful of how every biological function and instrument in our body is interrelated with the entire orchestra of our being. We can see how active children do not develop weight problems, or anger issues, and their spine is naturally healthy. Have you ever connected the kidney functions with the scoliosis of your child, or, the ulcer with the TV and its influence on the stomach, digestion and spine? Well, they certainly are connected, and it requires diligence on the parent's part to keep the child's health in good working order. My point is that it takes attention and balance to help our children keep their good health and balanced development. We must start to think about disease prevention rather than disease diagnosis and cure. There is no cure for any disease in the medicine bottle. I know that every one of us knows that fact already. But, the prevention is so easy, yet absolutely rewarding. Personally, I never had health insurance, and neither did any of my children. We prefer to see health as our biggest and most precious asset and responsibility, and save it that way. I would like to emphasize how important it is to develop and learn simple awareness. Yet, on the other hand, if a child gets severely ill, do not search for answers in my book, call your doctor. My book suggests how to keep healthy, for yourself and your child. Nevertheless, if you have not done it by now, and your child is sick, consult a doctor, you can get back to this book any time after the crisis is over, and start a systematic new way of awareness and health maintenance.

Chapter six
My little natural home pharmacy
This is the list of Homeopathic remedies, with suggested potency that I recommend having on hand at home, just in case.

- LM is a very high dilution and serves best but should not be repeated versus 6x which is a more crude dilution can be administered 3-5 times daily.

1. Arnica Montana 16 LM / 6x

2.Arsenicum Album 16 LM

3.Ac-Ph (Phosphoric Acetum) 6x

4.Belladonna 16 LM/ 6x

5.Gelsemium Sempervirens 16 LM/ 6x

6 Carbo Vegetabilis 16 LM/6x

7   Sulfur 16 LM /6x

8 .Rhus Toxicodendron 16 LM/ 6x

9.Nux Vomica 16 LM /6x

10. Pulsatilla Nuttaliana 16 LM /6x

11.Ignatia Amara 16 LM /6x

12.Natrum Muriaticum 6Lachesis 16LM /6x

14. Apis 16 LM/6x

15. Wasp 16 LM/6x

16.Calcarea Carbonica 6LM

17.Baryta Carbonica 16LM

18. Gluten 12X

19. Jalapa 16LM/6x

20. Formica Rufa 6X

21.Argentum Nitricum 16 LM

22.Ledum Palustre 16LM/6x

Giggling Dr. Green

23. Silicea 6X

Though it seems a very long list, and maybe a little costly up front, it is the best collection to have at hand at all times. Please compare this investment with the cost, and ineffectiveness of repeated doctor's visits, not to mention the inconvenience of bundling up an ill child, going out in the night and waiting goodness knows how long to be handed a prescription over and over again. Having all these remedies helped me raise five active children by keeping everything on hand that I needed to care for them in each and every case. Children certainly can get themselves into many unexpected situations, and having the right remedy, for the right condition, at the right moment is a sheer blessing and virtually priceless. It is not necessary to purchase the whole list at once. However, it is a very good idea to set it as an important goal. There are many simple ways to learn how to choose the right remedy for the right condition.

24. Apple Cider Vinegar (ACV) (more details can be found in chapter 10)

25. Tea Leaves and Seeds

Chamomile flowers, Mint leaves, Lavender flowers, Sage leaves, Rosemary leaves, Thyme, Parsley, Anise, Fennel Seeds, Caraway seeds, Hemp Seeds, flax seeds.

Ointments and Gels
Arnica Gel

Thuja cream

Graphites Cream

Hamamelis

Aloe Gel

Propolis

Tiger Balm

Eucalyptus Drops

Arnica Solution

Vitamin E liquid

Coconut oil

Honey

Egg white

Giggling Dr. Green

Other useful ideas for Home Pharmacy

Rolled Oats

Prunes

White Clay

Black tea and Chamomile tea bags

Hand Shower

Small bathing bowl for small children

Tweezers

Epsom Salt

Dead Sea Salt

Flax seeds

Small towels and cotton cloths

Dr. Shany DVD Reflexology course

Ear Candles

Suction cups

Cotton Balls

Warm water bottle (rubber bottle)

Infrared light.

****

This simple collection can help you treat your child and family for nearly any given problem. It can be crucial to have the best solution on hand. It should be all placed in one cool, well ventilated and neat place. This way you can easily find everything you need when you are under the stress of a crying or even screaming little child at 2 AM.

This is the time when we lose our ability to think clearly and easily forget where we put what. It would be very helpful to prepare a list, ahead of time, with the different names and different possible uses for each condition and complaint.

Keep in mind that everything that works for your child, would work as well for adults. Therefore, the investment is well worth it. Providing you are one of those who would go through any necessary effort just to avoid hospitals and unnecessary medications. Some of us live in remote areas and doctors are not so easy to reach. With Homeopathy, especially with these highly diluted remedies, you can address practically any problem without causing any harm. All those home pharmacy suggestions have absolutely no harmful side effects. Homeopathy works by the rule: "It is either all or nothing". In other words; if you happened to miss evaluate the situation, or your observation was not correct, no harm can be done with the wrong remedy choice. It can only be unsuccessful and would not give you the expected results. In this case, after waiting for an hour or, in case of emergency, 10 minutes, simply try a different remedy. This would also give you the time to call your Homeopathy practitioner and consult with him or her. To save the time to run and look for the pharmacy that might have that right remedy and the right dilution and the time to rush to the Homeopath is worth a million. It is different if all you need to do is make a phone call and get the suggestion for the right remedy.

Homeopathic remedies do not spoil with time as long as they are hidden from direct sun and the containers are tightly closed. Once a Homeopathic remedy has been touched, the dropper, the capsule or the pill, the whole batch is to be disposed of, or it will not work anymore. The reason is the highly diluted solution will "take on" any other "energy" message if contaminated this way.

When Jeff called me at 5 PM in Colorado, it was 1 AM his time in Europe. He was so grateful to have had the right remedy at hand, because his wife had severe food poisoning and they just arrived at the hotel. He was very grateful since he didn't know any doctor there. His only choice would be the emergency room which was very far from their hotel. This is not as serious, probably and not as stressful as with a little child. Between the little Homeopathy kit and my two hands for Reflexology, I counted my blessings to be always ready for any surprise. My children never went to the ER when they were ill. We always managed just by these very simple, harmless and efficient applications. I never gave my children any prescription medications.

The fact that a health problem is addressed right away, keeps it from deteriorating and complications. For example, when a child started a fever, lost his appetite, was grumpy with excessive thirst etc, the Reflexology and Homeopathy would alleviate the situation right away. (Ac-Ph would be my first choice or Aconitum) From that point on the child was never neglected, never had to wait in line at the doctor's office or be taken to the emergency room. Even a few days of high temperature is no reason to be alarmed, since the body has been supported in its battle to regain its healthy condition. Shay had severe dysentery when he was just 4 years old. The whole kindergarten was sick and all his friends had to be taken to the hospital. The real danger was dehydration because of the bloody diarrhea. Since he was so sick and could not drink which was so vital for his recovery, I simply poured water with a little bit of sea salt into his mouth with a teaspoon every minute. I administered Ars-A 16LM every 2 hours until he started to drink by himself. He thanked me as a little boy for not taking him to the hospital. Complications and deterioration occur most of the time from medications to lower the temperature or, to suppress the inflammation. These are the cases we hear about that can turn into adverse situations. It could be prevented if the body had just been supported. After all - disease indicates the battle of the body to recover health. The temperature indicates the activity of the white blood cells and the lymphatic cells. They increase like an addition of an army division when it is necessary. When the temperature is then unnaturally suppressed, it is as if the extra army division would be sent, yet unarmed. How would this division be able to help in combat? On the other hand, if we just cool off very gently the body's surface, meaning the skin, with wet towels, and/or Reflexology, in order to stimulate the circulation, the warm blood would then run back into the body slightly cooler and would help the child to fight the disease, rather than disarm the child. When disarming through fever suppressing medications, we actually put our child in great danger. The white blood cells as well as the lymphatic fluids cannot eradicate and consume the invading cells, whether there are viruses or bacteria. (The PH cannot be balanced back to the proper alkaline level it needs to be).

In the Homeopathy chapter, I will give you a few indications for each remedy. It would be a good idea to get familiar with it ahead of time, and maybe stick the simple guidelines on the inner door of your medicine cabinet for emergencies.

Definitions of Common complementary medicine Terms

Acute

Any ailment of short duration, such as infectious diseases, diarrhea, headache, vomit, sinus infection, skin rash or boil, etc. Acute ailments may become chronic if unresolved when the acute symptoms will be suppressed with anti- medications and the real cause will not be addressed and subsided. For example: children with recurring ear infections may get significant amounts of antibiotic medications. Unless you remove any dairy from their nutrition, and often gluten containing food, the ear infections will never stop. However, it is no secret that some antibiotic medications may lead to complications like, anxieties, nightmares, allergic reactions and even mental and emotional disorders that can turn even deadly. Insanity, leukemia, chrons, kidney failure and many more. I had never seen any complications of any kind by prevention of dairy, gluten and meat, yet). An acute ailment is self-limiting and of short duration; meaning it will usually run its course until recovery and strengthen the resistance. Acute disease is when the body displays all the signs of fighting such as, diarrhea, vomiting, fever, perspiration, mucus, discharges, rash, pain, pus, etc.

Aggravation

A noticeable increase in the severity of the disease symptoms previously observed. Sometimes associated with a temporary reaction of the body to the correct homeopathic remedy. Homeopathic aggravation would only be for a very short time, like minutes or an hour. It proves the choice of Homeopathic remedy to be the right one. The reason is: the body "displays" the symptoms of the "similar" disease and that disease helps the body to overcome the condition it got sick by. The "homeopathic disease" is actually only a mirror-image/mimic, of the real disease and lasts very short time, since it is just a message the cells received. This reaction provides the cells the time to; "learn how to deal" with the original condition and the healing process starts being effective.

Allopathic

The dominant medical system in the West, mainstream medicine that "fights" the disease instead of supporting the body - learn to fight. This is done by using the doctrine of opposites. (Antibiotics, antihistamines, anti-rash, anti-fungi etc,)

Antidote

A substance, treatment procedure, or a remedy, that counteracts the effect of a homeopathic remedy. For example, lemon, vinegar, ice, or black coffee can be used as an antidote for many homeopathic remedies in case of a more severe reaction. In most cases it could be a reaction that is found to be a little too harsh when the person is too weak to endure the healing process and needs more crude remedies) to a homeopathic remedy, an antidote may be given to neutralize the effects. (In case, too much homeopathy was applied or too crude of a dilution could also be the case, as all the 30C dilutions for example)

Cell Salts

W.H. Schuessler, a noted homeopathic physician, developed the Biochemical system using 12 different 'cell salts'. Dr. Schuessler felt these were fundamental to the proper function of the human body. Prepared in low potency,

Giggling Dr. Green

(3x or 6x), and used based on homeopathic indications. (Dr. Schuessler found the proper cell salts through his patients' astrology charts)

Characteristic Symptom modalities - are the key.

This describes a symptom, or group of symptoms, that is striking, strange, unusual, or peculiar in the case. Close attention is paid to characteristic symptoms, as they must correspond to symptoms of the remedy if it is to cure. (For instance, very high temperature, yet very big hunger. On the other hand, when he sees food, he loses the appetite. Alternatively, extreme thirst yet takes only tiny sips. Or, in extreme cold weather you have to kick the blanket off etc.) A well trained and experienced Homeopath will find those modalities through the answers to his questions.

Chronic

Meaning of long duration such as eczema or asthma or any illness and or disorder that lasts longer than three months. (Chronic ailments may have acute episodes, however) Chronic ailments are those that do not usually resolve of their own accord, when the patient does not display any "fighting" elements like those I mentioned at the acute symptoms. Unlike acute ailments.

Common Symptoms

These are symptoms that are common to a specific disease, for example, stiff joints with arthritis, or yellow skin with jaundice, fever and runny nose with flu, etc

Constitutional

Also known as 'classical', 'totality', 'Hahnemannian', 'Kentian', this means the remedy is prescribed for the perceived whole of the patient; includes symptoms and characteristics often with special attention to the emotional and psychological qualities. It is the epitome of 'Holistic' medicine. (Should always be the rule)

Electromagnetic Field

Healthy cells have a very different electromagnetic field than the unhealthy cells. This is what the immune system is all about. When our cells are healthy, that means that they have the absolute proper conditions, which are the worst conditions for every bacterium, virus, fungus and every cancer cell.

Homeopathy

A safe and natural method to restore the balance of body mind and spirit, and allow the body to heal and strengthen itself. Homeopathy stimulates the body's

Giggling Dr. Green

ability to heal with extremely highly diluted remedies prepared of natural substances. The beauty of homeopathic medicine is in its safety, the incredibly minute amount of remedy needed, and the rapidity of healing. The name; Homeopathy stems from two Greek words, (Homo; means like, Pathy; means heals. Like heals-like.) Homeopathy therefore means "similar cures similar" or "like cures like". Samuel Hahnemann, the founder of Classical Homeopathy, first coined the word Homeopathy.

LM

The second potency scale developed by Hahnemann, introduced in the sixth edition of the Organon. Start with a 3c triturate of a remedy. One part is placed into 500 drops of liquid (400 drops water, 100 drops alcohol). One drop is placed into 100 drops of alcohol. This is succeeded by hand 100 times. One drop of this mixture is used to medicate 500 #10 pellets. This is the Q1 potency, which is sometimes written as 0/1. The Q2 is made by taking 1 of these medicated pellets, putting it into 1 drop of water, and then mixing into 100 drops of alcohol. This mixture is succeeded 100 times by hand.

Today, the HPUS standard differs from Hahnemann's. Like Cures Like For example, if your symptoms are similar to poisoning by mercury, then mercury would be your homeopathic remedy. If your symptoms come from chocolate, the remedy should be chocolate in Homeopathic dilution. Omrie is very allergic to chocolate. When she was a toddler and went to daycare, she got a severe allergy attack. The teacher told the father who rushed to pick her up that she saw too late that Omrie received a chocolate chip cookie from her friend at lunch. In spite of the teacher's suggestion to rush Omrie to the emergency room, he called me telling me that he was heading my way and will be there in just 15 minutes. Omrie was wheezing and her eyes were shut red and tearing. I heard the story from her father on the phone, and took the chocolate remedy out. It was like a miracle. It took two seconds from the time the remedy touched Omrie's tongue and the attack was history.

Modality

This describes a condition that makes a person or their symptom better or worse. For example, better in a hot bath, abdominal pain, better bending over, worse in rainy weather, etc. Modalities are the most vital information for a complete symptom.

Mother Tincture

Giggling Dr. Green

The original standardized preparation of a substance from which homeopathic potencies are made.

Organon

The Organon of Medicine, by Samuel Hahnemann, the founder of homeopathy. This book describes the principles and practice of homeopathy. Hahnemann wrote six editions of the Organon from 1810-1842. The sixth edition, though finished in 1842, was not actually published until 1921. .

Potency

The strength of a homeopathic remedy. Determined by how many times the remedy has been succeeded and diluted during preparation. A number and a letter are associated with the remedy name to indicate which potency scale has been used. The three potency scales currently in use are decimal, centesimal and millesimal. An example of the decimal scale would be Arnica 6x.

An example of the centesimal scale would be Arnica 30c. (From my best mentor I learned never to use this potency.)

An example of the 50 millesimal scale would be Arnica LM1.

Potentized

This term usually refers to a substance prepared according to homeopathic pharmaceutical standards. This means that it has gone through serial dilution and succussion. (Like saying, "energized"). (For every Homeopathic remedy the succussion is the most important point)

Proving

The most accurate method of ascertaining the action of medicines on human health. Medicines, usually crude, are administered to healthy people to discover the symptoms they are capable of producing and with the potentization and dilution the symptoms subside.

Remedy

Medicine (Homeopathic medicine to name it differently from the medicine of the mainstream medicines), treatment, as in homeopathic remedy.

Vital Force, chi

The energy that maintains life in the individual., and every living creature and plant.

Giggling Dr. Green

Encounter with a Cactus

In 1976, my house was filled with children between the ages of 6 months and 10 years old. During that time, my husband was away for 30 days in the army for routine service duty. We were always prepared for the immediate draft of the army servicemen and women, at least, but not only, 30 days each year. They could be called for even longer, as the Army found it necessary, not including war times. At war times we never knew when our husband, son, brother or friend would return - if at all. The conditions in Israel were just a fact we learned to live with and not questioned. We were simply born into these conditions unfamiliar with any other reality. At the south of the Dead Sea small village and a house full of kids, I really felt as though we were living in the American Wild West, as seen in movies with Clint Eastwood or John Wayne. It simply was another fact in our daily life. Naturally, it forced us to be very creative in developing survival skills, to be assertive and tough that wouldn't be part of a normal urban woman's life. However, as I write this part, I realize that even now, war is in Iraq as well as in Afghanistan and a war ended not long ago in Sarajevo, and the war in Lebanon 2 summers ago. Therefore, I take my words half way back, because, sadly, there are many more places in which women have to develop those very important survival skills even today, and to never break down. Breaking down is not an option. It is a luxury we could not afford. I feel for all these women around the world in all the countries in war.

Yet, if, by any chance this book happens to reach you women, I pray that it will help you throughout those very worrisome, scary moments when there is no doctor to be found and your child gets sick. I wish to have the honor to be helpful and encouraging to all women who may have just these wild flowers in their backyard, or, the cold-water washes, or, maybe just a way to warm the potatoes to help alleviate the heavy cough of her child. For all of these women, I am writing this book. Before I continue I like to give you all a little important tip: If you don't have the needed homeopathic remedy, write it on a little piece of paper, hold it against the child's right side under the ribs, tap up and down the back, lightly and gently, up and down for about 10 times. Continue to hold this little note for a few more seconds. This will amaze you how wonderful it works.

At that time of adversity, as I was home alone with my little friends, Maayan played outdoors with her friends and law and behold, fell into a huge cactus bush. She came running home, screaming at the top of her lungs, because her body was covered with thorns. The baby was screaming because it was that time of the day, the 2 year old was suffering with severe bloody diarrhea, and the other two were fine, thank God. When Maayan came screaming I was at a loss for what to do. I did not know what else to do and I started pulling all the thorns out of her body. We had no car, and I did not even have a buggy or horse to get her to a doctor or emergency room. It was dawn and even the buses would stop only once a day, 8 miles away from our home. It was a real challenge and I was very young. God blessed me, as you already understand, with good ideas when I need them, and so, I decided that if I were to fill the bathtub with warm water, the skin pores would dilate and the thorns would simply fall out. And so it was. With no better idea, I put Maayan into the hot tub (not too hot of course) and let her body just "release" the thorns into the tub. It worked miraculously.

Today I still think that it is a great way to get thorns out of the skin, however, had I known better then, I would have given her a few pills of Silicea 6x, also. This miraculous remedy helps the body to "push out" foreign elements like thorns, splinters, etc. In those years, I had to learn firsthand to practice my Homeopathy and Natural Healing skills more than any apprenticeship I could ever get. The-learn as you go to school of natural medicine!

How to choose a Homeopathic remedy

Homeopathic remedies are not a big investment; however, they make a whole lot of a difference when needed. To look at our child's pain from a yellow jacket sting, and the right homeopathic remedy is at hand - is way more than sheer luck. It is heaven. Raising five children in the middle of the desert taught me to be organized and prepared for any unexpected and surprising new adventure with any one of them. I am sharing these little ideas with you and promise you; they will mean the world to you when the time comes to use them.

Suggestions; how to apply the Homeopathic remedies

1. **Arnica** 16 LM (Arn 16LM)

Arnica or named also Arnica Montana, a mountain plant commonly used in the relief of bruises, and muscle soreness. Arnica is widely used as a salve for bruises and sprains, and sometimes as a tincture, for the same anti-inflammatory, pain-relieving purposes. In homeopathy, it has a wider use;

This member of the sunflower family reminds us of cuts and bruises of all kinds.

Giggling Dr. Green

Arnica is considered also as a "surgical remedy" (even if the problem is violent anger).

The reason I prefer the drops is, because at times of pain, the child will not always cooperate when they are asked to open their mouth. Dropping the Homeopathic remedy into their little mouth, even when they are crying, always works.

In all cases of physical or emotional trauma, such as falls or accidents of any kind. Fractures, bruises, wounds, burns, cuts, or any violent experience. When the child is sick, and refuses to see the doctor to get help. For sunburn, burns from fire, and any kind of heat source. Lightening or frostbite. Any type of bites, including dog bites, cat bites and scratches. Outbursts of uncontrollable anger either by the child, or when the child was the victim of such. Everything that is connected with extreme pain and harmful conditions. Very high fever with restlessness and anger. After surgery, and 2-3 days before (if surgery had been scheduled.), tooth extraction. Thorns, mosquito bites.

2. **Arnica Gel**

It is also called Arniflora in some brands. Uses; all bruises, cuts, injuries, sunburns, cold sores, and scratches on the skin. It is good to administer in accordance with the intake of the Arnica drops, though it certainly is useful regardless of the drops. For external use only; red skin, scratched, bruise, burns, itch, hot, cold, freshly stitched. I could not consider my home injury safe without Arnica on hand.

3. **Arsenicum Album** 16 LM (Ars-A 16LM)

For the choice of this remedy, we need to remember the picture of an old, worried, weak and very pale man. It is an absolute must for any kind of poisoning or when the child looks as if he or she is about to pass out, or has passed out already. When the child is very pale; of fear, anxiety, shock, food poisoning, poisonous sting, severe diarrhea, or severe vomiting. When the child is thirsty, yet is able to take just very little sips. When the eyes look as if "a life threatening fear and very anxious", when the lips turn purple and the eyes display deep fear and when the threat is real. When the asthma attack is causing the eyes to bulge out with the fear of suffocation, when the child describes the pain as an unbearable burning sensation. When the child worries too much and is very sad and pessimistic. The general appearance is of a dry complexion, pale and sunken, as if very old. When the child's life is in danger of poisoning, suffocation, or alike, with significant restlessness. In cases of severe diarrhea vomiting, dehydration, extreme weakness, faintness and it looks as if the person lost his life force.

Giggling Dr. Green

4. **Belladonna** 16 LM (Bell 16LM)

Remember the bright red tongue, or burning red cheeks, or the very hot skin that cannot be ignored (once you touch the forehead or hand the heat stays for a long time in your hands memory). In an angry outburst, the face blushes to strawberry red, the mouth may drool, and the child can bite and tear everything apart.

This remedy has a few very easy indications, and helps very quickly when correctly chosen. Belladonna should not be given more than once or twice a day, and no longer than a week consecutively (I would use the LM dilutions only!). The indications for the choice of this remedy are Violence, very sudden, unexpected and extreme. The notion of; it happened "out of the blue" and then disappears, the same way. Or, when the child is waking up at night and suddenly screams as if something horrible has just happened as in screaming from nightmares. When a sharp and very sudden pain shoots through any part of its body and it screams so loud that you think a shark or lion is in its bed. When the fever appears so suddenly "out of the blue" yet, shoots sky high within minutes. When you touch the child, it feels so hot, that the warmth of that heat stays in your hand for quite a while. When the eyes, face, or any part of the body is extremely hot, bright red, extremely painful and swollen. Belladonna symptoms appear very unexpected, fast, violent, extreme, burning pain, and so bad that you may consider rushing your child to the ER.

Belladonna helps when any organ is swollen like a bag full of fluid, and Belladonna helps to "empty" these swelling fluids. Belladonna helps also when the child is too giggly and can't stop, when the child has an aversion to water, or feels panicky especially around water, when the reflection of any shiny object or water causes the attack or convulsions and seizures, when the child is very violent and when angry gets extremely red in eyes and face, rips things apart. When the complaint is; "like pins and needles", or; "tiny thorns in the skin".

In many cases, extreme violence is not to be overlooked. Belladonna people can be dangerous.

Also helpful in case of dog bite, especially in case of a bite with rabies.

Any brain inflammation, meningitis or severe sudden impacting headaches, gallbladder attacks, uterus pain at menstrual cycle or ovarian pain; "feels like filled with fluid and about to burst", bladder infection, when the mouth saliva is drooling and eyes are bulged and breathing is heavy and difficult.

Giggling Dr. Green

Remember; any sour food or drink can make things worse. So does cold water or ice. For liver and gallbladder, the Belladonna is very calming as well. Please use it only in acute cases. For lingering problems Belladonna will not work, and Calc-C should be considered to replace Belladonna.

When Tom told me his embarrassing problem, he seemed to feel lost and could not find help anywhere. He told me how he would scream at night in his sleep, and would not even wake up. He was helped after just two doses of Belladonna 18 LM.

When Eli was having asthma attacks and had no medication to help, he came to me with his aunt. She told me that he gets the most violent anger attacks, and it does not matter what the trigger may be. They felt helpless at home and feared his attacks. His saliva would drool and his eyes looked as if about to pop out of their sockets. He was very upset with me when I said that his asthma was not his lungs problem, but his anger, and the cause would be in his liver and kidneys. He was in his teens and facing the fact that he was not as sick physically as much as he was in a vicious out of control anger cycle, did not make him very happy, regardless of my explanations.

Belladonna helped to calm him down, get more control of his anger and eventually stopped the asthma attacks.

5. **Gelsemium** 6LM (Gels 6LM)

Remember the condition when the "head feels too heavy to lift off the pillow". Diarrhea comes on suddenly, from fright, bad news: the stool will be involuntary. The child has a sudden, intense fear of falling down or fainting if asked to stand up. Cold and flu symptoms may be present; the child describes her head as being so painful she cannot lift it off the pillow. When the child who is fully bathroom trained, cannot hold his bladder, especially if you are aware the problem began when the child received a sad or worrisome message. When speech is unclear, reading, and writing are a problem.

When fear and vertigo are part of the complaints.

When falling asleep is a problem that does not find a solution, and sleepless nights are just a given.

Gelsemium I would use for most of the unbearable headaches, when the feeling of faintness is present, after a phone call that "changed" the child's life.

Migraine headaches, all the sphincters are in distress when Gelsemium is needed. You can see it in the pupils, when the stomach feels as if the "entrance is tied with a string", when the throat feels like it will close all together, when the

Giggling Dr. Green

vocal cords "skip" a tone. The Gelsemium is a treasure to have at your reach when there is any tendency to stress related constrictions, constipation and everything else you can imagine that can feel tight after bad news. I treated a woman with devastating headaches for 50 years that no homeopath succeeded to heal. All I got from her story was, "I remember my first devastating migraine headache after hearing my mother saying very alarming things on the phone, and did not realize that I was listening. It never went away." One dose of Gelsemium 16 LM did the trick. The migraines never re-occurred.

When Sam had his learning difficulties, he was treated for a while with Gelsemium, which helped him to focus and control his eliminations and his speech improved significantly.

Sara was a veterinarian who suffered from insomnia for many years. When taking her Homeopathic picture I learned that it started after her mother called her one night, right before she was ready for bed. Gelsemium 18 LM helped her after only 3 applications.

6. **Carbo Vegetables** 16LM (Carb-V 16LM)

When the child is weak, dehydrated or has diarrhea and the lips are purplish or surrounded by a pale circle. When the child got sick in a tropical location, where there was high heat and humidity, he was too weak to get up. When the child is weak from diarrhea or/and fever or profuse perspiration. It helps the body to better absorb oxygen. It is probably the best reviving remedy.

7. **Sulfur** 16 LM (Sulf 16LM)

When the skin, the hair, the bedroom, clothes, and even the child or the wound look dirty and filthy, or if filth was the trigger. For all infectious diseases that are connected with filth and hygiene deficiency. When the cough is and sounds wet, or dry. When the child has a boil, or when the rash seems to have pus in it. When perspiration, breath, feet, hair, stools and even burps smell like sewer, real foul smell. Even the skin looks as if it was never washed. Everything in a person that smells foul and bad.

A good counteracting remedy for all suppressed diseases, like through antibiotics, and vaccinations. Significant dryness and thirst are typical for Sulfur. When the child gulps water like it had never done before.

I would start any condition of infection with huge thirst with or without fever, with Sulfur. You can never go wrong with Sulfur.

Giggling Dr. Green

In many cases, the emotional and or mental picture would "look" exactly like the physical picture, and the choice would be the same. (Like results of suppressed anger, sadness etc.)

With aravens hunger, however, when the child sees the food, the appetite is lost.

<u>Please note</u>: When applying sulfur and an old forgotten disease "shows up", do not get alarmed. It is a typical quality of sulfur, and is the best way to treat chronic diseases. Also, when the gas or stools smell like rotten eggs, sulfur would be the remedy of choice.

Excellent remedy to counteract and neutralize vaccines side effects and damage.

8. **Rhus Toxicodendron** 16 L (Rhus-T 16LM)

Reminds you of a poison ivy rash. It is helpful for all skin problems that resemble poison ivy.

Key word for Rhus –T would be "too". Too much of anything.

Extreme restlessness and the need for a hard surface to lie on.

When children are over exposed to stress, sun, cold, physical activity, joint pain, muscle soreness, restlessness, pain that gets better with activity yet worse after rest and first thing in the morning. When the child feels better lying and sitting on hard and straight surfaces such as the floor instead of the bed or couch, or sitting on a wooden bench instead of on a soft chair.

When children are very angry and are suffering from the results of their anger (like backache, wrist pain, stomach ache and even headache). When warmth alleviates the suffering. Symptoms become worse from cold, and softness. It is in many ways a little bit like Arnica, but it does not work as well for acute problems, and much better for more lingering problems. Skin rashes can be helped tremendously with Rhus-tox, if the reason for the rash is stress, anger, dairy and cold. Rhus-Tox rash is very itchy, and looks like a collection of very small pimples or grain-like acne heads. Unlike the Belladonna, the Rhus-tox complaints come slowly and disappear slowly

9. **Nux Vomica** 16 LM (Nux-v 16LM)

(The common name of Vomiting Nut explains it all.)

It works like magic in so many cases that you can almost not go wrong using it. For contagious diseases, virus transmitted flu and colds, upset stomach, sore back and muscles, after antibiotics, and can undo the side effects of many medications such as sedating medications, pain-killer medications, narcotic medications, caffeine related or any symptoms resembling irritability. Night hunger, diarrhea. Constipation in which you can see the child needs to go but cannot empty his bowels enough. Anger related complaints, but here it is more anger due to a competitive personality that cannot take defeat. Food poisoning that leads to diarrhea and vomiting. Over eating, that makes your child feel as if the food has not moved the right direction. The most interesting indication for Nux-V is the good appetite in spite of the disease, and the child feels much better after eating.

10. **Apis** 15LM (Apis 15LM)

When thinking of Apis, just think of everything you know about honeybees. Apis is made from bees. If a bee stung your child, Apis would be the best choice. There is Apis ointment available as well as Apis caplets and a liquid form. Apis helps with mosquito bites if Arnica does not do the job. Apis will work wonders when a child is screaming from the top of its lungs and it sounds like a shriek that pierces all the way through your bones.

For urinary tract complaints such as burning when urinating, or frequent urination with sharp pain. When the kidneys are involved and there is already swelling in the face or joints. So, when children suffer from all kinds of joint inflammation. When the child is very restless and looks like a bee that is zooming around very restlessly. When the child prefers warm temperatures yet, the shower feels better with cooler or even cold water.

WARNING! Never give a child a cold bath, even if their temperature seems alarming. In an Apis child it can cause convulsions and may be life threatening. So, even if the child loves cold water, do not put it into a cold bathtub. Only-warm **NOT** hot and not cold!

Apis works miracles in many skin rashes, because the skin is considered in complementary medicine as "the third kidney". It makes a lot of sense when you think about it. When the kidney, for any reason, cannot flush out all the toxins that it needs to in order to preserve life, the next organ would be the skin. We see the rash and know how hard the kidney tries to release all these toxins and how potent they are, so they "attack" the skin. In other words, it would be wise to use Apis because it helps the kidneys to deal with toxins, and the rash will disappear when the kidneys are well.

When administering Apis, do not use any additional bee products, such as honey, propolis, or bee pollen.

Giggling Dr. Green

All eye infections, red eye, swollen eyes, irritated eyes, itchy eyes, sore throat, after colds and flu.

11.**Ignatia Amara** 16 LM (Ign A 16LM)

Excellent when the grief is lingering, feeling of guilt is paralyzing. Ignatia Amara is a remedy of grief and guilt, common among artists, hysteria, and inconsolable weeping.

When a cough gets worse, and the more she coughs the stronger the cough gets. When she cries she will increase the sobbing when you try to console. Constipation and rectal complaints. When the child feels like "a furry ball is stuck in the throat" or a knot in her stomach. When the child is very artistic and only expresses its feelings through its art. When knee pain "jumps" to the wrist, or to the shoulder or heel. When Tonsillitis repeats itself after the child suffers a painful separation and loss. When the child has a complaint of a "ball stuck in its throat" with tonsillitis, constipation, or any other pain, or even outbreak. Winy and inconsolable. When the child feels regret for something it had done and wished he had not done it. Even when the symptoms seem like virus or bacteria caused, and they accompany the previous emotional problem. Ignatia is a remedy of remorse, regret, guilt, shame, that presents itself in the physical body more than any other disease. Like warts on the skin that do not respond to any skin treatment - Ign will help if you find the reason behind any of the previously mentioned emotions.

12.**Pulsatilla** 16 LM (Puls 16LM)

This is for when the child who used to drink water suddenly claims he is not thirsty and is very cuddly, wanting to be held much more than normally.

When a child is sick with a high fever, in very warm weather and you have tried everything to get her to drink something, yet she continues to refuse, saying she is not thirsty.

The child in need of Pulsatilla feels much better even in very cold weather when you take it outside. When the complaints are at "both ends of the body, up and down". For example, when the throat hurts and the foot also, and for when the child perspires only on one side of the body. The child needing Pulsatilla gets very sick after eating dairy, baked goods, shellfish and pork.

A Pulsatilla child is the easiest, most loving and appreciative patient.

Gets easily sick from wind, cold water. Feels better when drinking cold water, even if getting sick from getting wet. When the ears ooze brown fluid after vaccinations.

Giggling Dr. Green

A great " vaccination neutralizing" remedy.

13. **Calcarea Carbonica** C12 (Calc-C 12C)

When the fontanel bones seem to be taking too long to close, Calc-C 12 is made in the center of the oyster shell, promoting the development of these bones. In addition, when the head is relatively big. When there are "egg" like swellings that feel like eggs or like marshmallows. The Calc-C is very important for children with a delay in their bone structure and fusion. It is the next step when Belladonna is needed but the problem takes a longer time, and the Calc-C takes longer to show results.

Calc-C, is very helpful to address results of anger yet the person is much less aggressive than the Belladonna anger.

When the joints hurt, when restlessness at night keeps the child up. When the child feels as if it needs structure in life and can't get it. This child bounces off the walls, is restless and "hard to control".

14.**Lachesis** 16 LM (Lach 16LM)

When the child is so talkative it seems he never stops talking. When there are noticeable purplish spots under the skin that seem like dark purplish bruises. Jealousy appears to be a major issue that truly controls his or her life and behavior.

Lach is a great remedy for all poisonous bites that resemble snake bites. When the nerves appear paralyzed and when the blood is poisoned. Like when sepsis conditions. When the blood consistency starts to deteriorate like in leukemia and anemia in blood cancer. Lach is a blood poison remedy and serves in cases of spider, snake, bullfrog or any venomous bites and exposures. It is necessary to have this remedy in every home. When the child has attacks as if it is suffocating and complains that it feels like their rib cage is closing in. When a child feels and describes he feels confined and trapped. When the child displays symptoms as if it were intoxicated by alcohol or recreational drugs.

When the child has inflamed tonsils, sore throat, yet feels better when swallowing something big that "feels as if it swipes the throat". Remember the picture of a snake that swallows prey much bigger than it seems it could? This is typical for lachesis. Feels much better when it is very warm. The skin may even peel like the snake's skin.

Heart issues, cough, anxiety, shock, poison, choking, etc. All could respond very well to Lach. Fear of bad dreams will create bedtime problems. Fear of death. Dreaming of lions, tigers, bears and snakes. Can't go to sleep for fear of the next morning, the time everything feels worse.

15.**Wasp** 16 LM (Wasp 16LM)

When stung by a wasp or any other similar insect. When the sting feels like a stab. When stabbed by any sharp object that is very painful. Every painful thorn poking the skin and causes severe pain with redness and swelling. Wild bees, wasps, yellow jackets, scorpions, spiders etc.

16.**Baryta Carbonica** 16 LM (Bar-C 16LM)

When the child displays development problems like dwarfishness of any kind. When the development is late. When any organ, hands, feet, are late in developing to the proper proportion, and seems way too small. It can be any function and any part of the physical or mental being. It seems too small.

In many cases of autism of any stage, it can do wonders. Yet, it is not an overnight remedy. It must be administered for a long time, dilutions in the LM's and not more than once a week.

17.**Gluten** 12X

For children who have different complaints specifically after eating any kind of baked goods. In addition, children who have been diagnosed with gluten intolerance and had any kind of wheat and or gluten food. In cases of unexplained diarrhea that keeps coming back even if there is no evidence for anything else that could be the reason.

For children with restlessness, (much better than medications like Ritalin), or those who have ADD, ADHD, difficulties learning reading and writing, are sensitive and easily get tonsillitis and or ear infections. If the remedy makes any impression on the child, prevention of any wheat and gluten must be kept very religiously.

18. **Jalapa** 16 LM (Jala 16LM)

This is a remedy for baby colic or when a child is very sensitive to any kind of spiced food.

19.**Formica Rufa** 6X (Form-R 6x)

The best remedy for any kind of ant bites, but especially for red ants' bites. Red ants are known to be extremely poisonous and some people would suffer severe swelling from their bites. This remedy can even save life in case of allergic reaction to ant bites, especially if there are more than one.

Giggling Dr. Green

20.Argentum Nitricum 16 LM

In cases of anxiety and when the imagination is confused with reality. For example, when the child describes how the buildings are touching each other at the top and is very scared.

When the child can see only "danger" in everything he is about to try or do, the child is fearful of anything. Fear of riding the car, fear of flying, fear that someone is out there to get him, fear of anything that keeps the child nervous with stomach pain and sweat. The child gets sick with fear. In many cases this remedy would work very well in accordance with Gelsemium.

21.Ledum 16 LM (Led 16LM)

Ledum serves as a first aid remedy for any injury, when the bleeding does not seem to stop fast enough and when internal hemorrhage is suspected. For bruises, falls, cuts, trauma, or any accident, Ledum will be helpful. (Like Arnica)

22.Silicea 6X (Sil 6X)

Silicea helps for mental exhaustion. When a child has just had too much stress and is very ambitious about grades, making the team. When unable to manage the daily simple tasks he had done before, he feels so exhausted. Everything is too overwhelming for him now. Best remedy for mental and academic exertion. This remedy is also a thorn and splinter pusher. When given after any invasion of any foreign object, the body will actually push it out. See the story about Maayan falling into the Cactus bush.

When Maayan tried to change the picture frames and opened the frame, the glass popped and a splinter flew right into her eye. She was old enough to suggest that we drive her to the emergency room. I thought it was better than trying anything else, since after all it was her eye, and I don't fumble around in eyes. After sitting and waiting in line for a whole hour, I suggested trying Silicea. The pain was really annoying and the line in the ER did not move. So we returned home and I administered Maayan 4 little globules of Silicea. It took 30 minutes when Maayan came down and showed me a pretty large sized splinter that she just felt coming out of her eye. This remedy is also amazing when the child gets any kind of splinters or nails.

23.Chamomile 16 LM (Cham 16LM)

Chamomile is a "natural antibiotic" and many times gets impressive results.

Giggling Dr. Green

It is especially recommended for fever, ear aches, stomach ache, and diarrhea, reluctant and resents any treatments or help. When a child gets very wild when you try to change its diapers, dress it, or even offer food. This remedy works like magic for these little rebels. Chamomile tea is also highly recommended, but you must not over use it because it will turn around and have the opposite effects when over used. However, with the highly diluted remedy, you may give it once or twice daily for two to three days and it is all right.

It should be in any household. For babies with colic or teething it works great.

Of course Chamomile is a great remedy for all ages.

24. **Aconite** 6x (Acon 6X)

At the onset of any fever disease. It is helpful to "stop" it or at least take the aggression out of any upcoming trouble. And it is still not suppressive like medications. Aconite just supports right from the start.

25. Thuja 6LM (Thuj 6LM)

Thuja helps to neutralize adverse side effects of vaccines. After Tetanus shots Thuja should be administered as well as after any vaccine. Thuja helps even after a significant time of the shots.

These are the most important remedies I would keep at reach for just in case. With this collection, every parent is prepared if anything happens at home or outdoors and the doctor's help is still far, or preferably avoided. When G.D was so sick and suffered from advanced Meningitis, his parents refused to take him to the Emergency Room. When they described his high fever and stiffness, I insisted on rushing him to the emergency room. "But what would you give him until we get there?" the father asked. Considering the circumstances under which he got sick, I would give Ars-A16 LM and *Belladonna* 18 LM to help reduce the swelling of the brain fluids. They had the remedies at home and applied them. He got so fast that they decided, against my suggestion, to continue the homeopathic remedies, and stay away from the hospital. I did not agree and felt that was a very irresponsible decision, which endangered the child. Thank God, he recovered. Please, do not take chances with your child in severe cases, consult a medical doctor.

Important note! I never intend to convince you not to take your child to the Emergency Room and/or doctor in case of such a severe illness. All I say is that, if you cannot get to the hospital, for any reason like a snow blizzard or a sand storm, or a truly wicked weather, or if there is no hospital in the area or you cannot get there, there are ways to help the child stay alive until you CAN get the medical help she or he requires. Please, in serious cases like those I mentioned above; do not experiment on your child like G.D. 's parents dared to do. He is lucky to be alive. Be wise and thoughtful, after all it is your dearest one's very life at stake.

These recommendations are only for cases when we want to help our child to overcome simple diseases, children illnesses, development concerns, acute and chronic illness and know that it is not of a life-threatening nature. Homeopathy can do wonders, indeed. Yet, it takes a very well trained and skilled Homeopath to make the proper choice in serious cases. These are just suggestions in case there is no other choice available. Moreover, for those of you who know their children very well and want to go the natural healing way, medication and invasive applications are free - keep them safe. If you do not know, ask. Call. Pre-educate yourself.

More helpful items for your home pharmacy

1. White Clay

White Clay is renowned for its internal and external health promoting properties and uses. Internally it helps to balance acidic stomach and digestive problems. Unfortunately, many children suffer from medications and chemotherapy side effects. For them white clay is very helpful. The external use of white clay is recommended in cases of red skin rash, boils, mosquito bites, and every closed skin inflamed condition. When the skin has not broken, yet it is swollen, hot and painful. It is very helpful when applied on a painful inflamed joint as well. It has the quality to "pull out" the inner heat and inflammation. Since these are not emergency conditions, yet still pretty painful, treat the child with white clay instead of any "anti inflammatory" over the counter medications. They never support the self healing mechanism but create nasty side effects and should definitely be avoided. Recent research and statistics show that the second cause of death in the US after accidents are the over the counter medications. Let us help our child not even look that way and begin with natural healing and only if it does not solve the problem, consult a trustworthy caring physician.

When Shay was stung by a wasp at the age of 4, white clay was the only "help" I had available in 2 minutes. It is the Dead Sea soil. I stuck his little finger in the wet soil and the pain was gone before it even began to swell.

After the 6 days war the "Jericho fly" started to be a health and beauty hazard in the Dead Sea vicinity, we were unfamiliar before. It was triggered by a fly bite that would leave a scar for the rest of your life. The wounds would last for many months, as the larva would develop under the skin and would require many months of antibiotic treatments, along with ointments and at times, even surgical procedures. This is via allopathic medicine. I found a miraculous remedy for it that would shorten the whole problem to just a few days. By mixing white clay with Apple Cider Vinegar and applying a generous "pile" on the wound, cover it with a wet cloth and keep the place in a restful position for 20 minutes. When I took it off, the little "pile" was like a small bowl filled with pus and the wound healed immediately after it. In the South of The Dead Sea, people were very apprehensive at first; yet, it worked like a miracle, without the need for any additional medications or surgery, of course. Needless to mention how no scars remained either.

2. **Rubbing Alcohol**

For external use only, the rubbing alcohol serves many purposes. It helps to disinfect any tool we may need to touch a wound. It helps to disinfect even the comb when we have to "fight" lice, reduces body temperature when the child runs a fever. Simply wet a small personal towel and apply it on the child's ankles and wrists. Be very careful not to come near the eyes and mouth.

When we have to pull a thorn out of our kid's skin, or a piece of glass it stepped on, we may want to clean the area and the tweezers before and after the "procedure". It is very important to keep everything very clean under any circumstances when we treat children.

3. **Olive Oil**

Oddly yet still a fact, olive oil has numerous health promoting properties that are very useful for our kid's health.

For dry skin, better than any scented and perfumed cream or lotion. Just a little olive oil diluted in warm water. Your child's skin will heal fast and well. For skin rash or eczema, constipation and dry stools, apply a little olive oil to the rectum, (instead of all the harmful cortisone creams). It does not slow the healing process; yet, it will help true healing versus superficial healing with harmful side effects and complications.

Olive oil is good for psoriasis. The olive oil stimulates the skin to actually heal itself. Seborrhea of the scalp. After you shampoo their hair, apply a little olive oil on the scalp and massage it lightly. It helps to rebalance the scalp and the seborrhea will disappear.

Reduces high cholesterol and triglycerides. A teaspoon of olive oil in their vegetable salad will help the body to clean their arteries. The olive oil helps the brain, nerve tissue, intestinal healthy activity, blood vessels, prevents possible complications resulting from high cholesterol and triglycerides. Olive oil helps to remove tar that sticks to the feet on certain beaches. Olive oil enriches the body with vitamin A+D, as well as Omega 3.

In the Mediterranean countries, olive oil is of great use. These countries enjoy a relatively low rate of heart diseases as well as liver and gallbladder disorders. Olive oil is vital for internal and external use. It helps to prevent constipation, and is very helpful when healing sunburn. Just one little drop into the ear canal, and the pain is gone. When heated, olive oil will not turn into saturated fat. For that, it needs much higher temperatures than the cooking temperatures we use. Olive oil is in every aspect the absolute and complete opposite of - Trans fats.

*Coconut oil can be used for the same purposes

4. EMFor brational medicine

Every atom in the Universe has a frequency, whether it is a rock, a drop of water or our own cells. Each cell resonates and vibrates at a specific frequency that is its own kind. Our body consists of a variety of atoms, which contain protons, electrons & an overall Bio Electromagnetic energy field that runs through it. The way we take care of our body physically, emotionally and mentally determines how our electromagnetic field resonances. This is the indication for health or, if the resonance is disturbed, disease.

The Electromagnetic Field device is best used regularly, twice daily in order to help the body keep the cells in good resonance and balance the healthy cell's electromagnetic field. A well-researched device helps to maintain a well functioning immune system. Helps to restore a damaged and poor immune system, regenerate organs and tissues, enhances the proper metabolism of the healthy cells, and helps the body to heal itself. The device is available in many countries as well as in America, and is very important equipment in every household for better fitness and health. Unlike any other mainstream medicine method, it is absolutely non-invasive, has no unwanted side effects and is very simple to use by every family member. This system is replacing a good workout, as well as helps in weight problems.

Nadav has used it since he was born, and knows how to push the buttons. It is based on Quantum Physics and is an energy differing and balancing tool for health and well-being. In many researches around the world, it has proved to enhance bone density, bone fusion and regeneration, besides the energy enhancement and health regeneration over all.

5. Apple Cider Vinegar

Giggling Dr. Green

Apple Cider Vinegar is considered in traditional natural therapy as the all in one, pharmacy in a bottle. It is very useful indeed for almost all problems. Some of them I will list here, and many of these secrets you can try yourself because it is absolutely healthy and has no harmful side effects. Just one precaution I would suggest – never come close to the eyes with the Apple Cider Vinegar. (Note! It is not FDA approved as a medicine.)

Therefore, here are some applications you can use for your child:

(When my grandchildren were infested with lice my choice was always to massage the Apple Cider vinegar diluted in water. To cool down the high temperature add a cup of Apple Cider Vinegar into the tab. Alcohol has been for me mainly for disinfection and far from children. It is recommended by many other Naturopathic practitioners though)

1) **Stomach** ache when the reason could be indigestion or gas. Use 1 tsp of ACV in 4-ounce water, mix with a little honey and let the child drink it slowly. When prepared correctly it is even very tasty.

2) **Diarrhea** can be treated the same way like as in #1, but could be served more than just once. Until the diarrhea subsides.

3) **Skin Rash** - use 1 tsp of ACV in 2-ounce water, dip a cotton ball into the solution, and tap the irritated skin area. It not only helps to calm it down, but helps the body to heal. You can put Apple Cider Vinegar in the bathtub and let the child sit in it. By helping to balance the PH, the skin heals and calms.

4) *Acne and Seborrheah*- (usually for older children but, not exclusively, could occur in babies as well) Use the same solution as #3, the same way on the irritated areas, a few times a day. Drinking the ACV (diluted and sweetened with honey!) in these cases helps the body to neutralize the PH and the skin will be less oily, so that will lift off the problem from the inside as well.

5) **Lice** – many children suffer from this easily transmitted problem in warm countries especially. After each shampooing rinse the head with the same solution like #1 and leave it in. Helps to get rid of lice as well as prevent the problem. Not all kids get lice and the reason for it is – the scalp acidity. This treatment balances the PH and helps your child not only against the lice, but also heal the scalp, hair and add a lot of shine to the hair. (Parents should use it too, since it helps reduce hair loss and improves hair condition)

6) **Flu and colds** – When the fever is high and the child gets the solution like #1, it helps the body to heal much faster. To soak in a tub with ACV added,

helps to feel much better faster, and the healing process gets easier and quicker. (The reasoning is the same as I mentioned before regarding the PH balance)

7) *Ulcers* of the digestive tract – several times a day, drinking the #1 solution before all meals, or, 40 minutes after each meal, helps the body to heal gastric ulcers. The reasoning is – The body creates ulcers when the very delicate inner linings of the stomach and intestines suffer from over acidity and insufficient enzymes. It also loses the positive micro flora vital for the autoimmune system as those produce the Vitamin B12 in the intestines. If the child gets excessive processed food, or not enough fresh fruits and vegetables, the inner linings begin to break into little sores, which develop into ulcers. The mainstream medicine claims the ulcers are due to bacteria, (which is true, but the only way to heal the body of bacteria is - not providing the bacterium fertile ground to thrive) and so prefer to treat ulcers with antibiotics, and so the ulcers actually never heal. The truth is, had the food been more alkaline producing, the bacteria would not be able to exist in the stomach in the first place. Fighting it with antibiotics or any other drugs will only turn it into a chronic drug dependent disease, which could easily evolve into cancer after a few years. The ACV replenishes the positive bacteria, creates an alkaline environment, serves as enzymes, and the body can heal completely. Kids after chemotherapy treatments may also suffer from the same problem, and should be given this wonderful drink.

8) *Nausea* - and over all upset stomach from overeating – Very small amounts of solution #1 until the child feels better, or throws up.

9) *Bulimia and Obesity* – A glass of solution #1 right before any meal and snack, will help the child to have the right enzymes to break down and digest the food it is about to eat. It also reduces hunger. Hunger is many times a sensation because of over acidity in the stomach rather than need for nutrition. It is a warning sign for developing ulcers or gastritis.

10) *Overweight* - even babies can suffer weight control problems, yes, kids that are hooked on soda pop, sugar rich beverages, as well as junk snacks may need the ACV to prevent clogging of their arteries, liver problems and weight control problems. For these reasons, I would recommend the #1 solution before and right after snack consumption.

11) *Kidney problems* – Like the other suffering organs, the kidney is also very burdened by the wrong nutrition for children. ACV helps to dissolve calcium deposits and fat molecules in the blood and therefore kidneys as well. Ph balancing with the ACV could avoid most of the related problems. Use the solution #1 at least 3 times daily.

Giggling Dr. Green

12) ***Gum disease, gingivitis and cavities*** - The source for these problems is like in all the other parts of the digestion problems. Bleached and artificial acid producing foods as well as sugar. Gurgling with solution #1 after each meal is significantly more helpful and efficient than using toothpaste. The toothpaste is actually solving only the industry's problem as to where to dump the toxic fluoride; they cannot dump it openly into the water. Therefore, they dump it into the toothpaste and poison not only the adults who could choose not to use it, but also for children who have to use it, because mom and dad said so as they do not know any better. Therefore, if you truly love your child, keep the toothpaste out of reach and start using the ACV solution instead. It will help to heal the gums, stop the mouth bad odor, help regain the balanced acid and alkaline in the mouth, and so prevent cavities and gum problems.

13) ***Tonsillitis -*** Gargling with ACV solution when the tonsils are swollen and red would be a much healthier and solving method than antibiotics. Every doctor knows by now that the antibiotics do not work anymore. The biggest fear of the Health Administrations all over the world is that within 5 years no drug and medicine will combat any inflammations disease and will have absolutely no effect on the bacteria, and will save not even one life if needed. So, if it is not helping anyways, why not take something so simple and healthy, that does work? If the child has inflamed tonsils or infected tonsils, help it by letting it drink very slowly ACV solution #1, as well as, if possible, gargling with it every 2 hours. It is healthy, the body will heal itself, and it is safe. It is also strengthening the soft tissue of the tonsils, while neutralizing the environment and helping the child simply get better and stay better. Remember the stories about these poor little kids who died because their body broke down from too much and too often antibiotics? Why put your child in danger? Not using antibiotics, letting the fever be and just supporting the course of the disease is absolutely your kid's lifesaver. To wrap a cloth or sock wetted with the ACV around the hurting neck will do wonders for your child.

14) ***Athlete's foot***/eczema- Soak feet once a day in a bowl with water, 3 Tbsp ACV and 1 Tbsp sea salt. Keep feet dry and change socks twice daily. Stop using detergents; wash the child's laundry with citrus vinegar only. Keep the child free of bleached flour and sugar products as well as dairy.

15) ***Sinus infection and headaches***- ACV drinks 3-4 times a day will help to neutralize the blood to become more alkaline and the body will fight these ailments much easier and faster. (Cold washings work well together with this recommendation)

Giggling Dr. Green

Keep a dairy free diet.

16) *Constipation*- 1 glass of ACV first thing in the morning as well as two more times a day will help to replenish the positive bacteria in the intestines, and will help the healthy blood and lymphatic fluid flow, to activate the bowel peristaltic activity and the child will heal itself.

Big orchard farmers who had to keep healthy throughout the winters when there were no fresh fruits or vegetables to be found first produced ACV in Europe.

The idea came from Dr. Gervis, who found that the fermented apples hold significant health promoting ingredients such as Kaolin, which is such a vital mineral for the digestion system and helps as an enzyme. The acidophilus that is produced by the fungus that creates the fermentation. The pectin in the apple is known to be vital and helpful for the immune system. The fact that the longer the ACV stays, the better it becomes. These are just a few of the ACV healing assets that no medication can beat.

I highly recommend keeping a bottle of ACV at home, and even in your travel bag. There is nothing too serious the ACV cannot help. On trips and camp outs it is a miracle in action.

Keep in mind, always to dilute it so it will never be used too strongly.

Did I mention that it helps lose weight and clean the arteries of plaque?

6. *Boric Acid* - Always good to keep at reach for small eye irritations (this is a solution and not a Homeopathic remedy)

7. *Enema*

Very helpful in cases of constipation, ear and sinus infections. A small lukewarm enema can relieve earache as well as sinus problems. It is based on the same logic as the cool washes of the private areas, or, putting cool, wet socks on the feet when ears ache.

8. *Honey*

Honey is a very helpful remedy for burns, (egg white should be added after the honey) wasp and bee stings. Honey, when served in small quantities, will aid in relaxation and calm down the restless child.

Honey has a significant beneficial impact upon the Autoimmune System. It is so powerful that it was found in Archeological findings without spoiling even after 3000 years.

9. ***Edible Castor Oil*** -When mixing 2 teaspoons of this oil with 3 tsp apple cider vinegar in a cup of honey, it serves as the best soothing and calming cough syrup. Syrup without harmful narcotic ingridients, unlike on the pharmacy shelves. This syrup is not suppressing the cough, but causing the phlegm to be coughed out in one good short cough, clearing the air pipes off flegm. The irritated throat will get the "opportunity" to calm down, yet the cough will still clean the airways and bronchi. For the expected results, serve 6 small spoons throughout the day if possible.

10. ***Epsom Salt-*** Useful for all sorts of stressful conditions and skin irritations, colds, stress, etc, in a bathtub. When feet hurt, athlete's foot or any skin irritation, when the overall feeling is inadequate. Pour a little Epstein salt into the water, and the child will soon feel much better.

11. ***Prunes-*** Always recommended to have on hand, either for constipation, as a very mild and painless bowel stimulator, or as a healthy snack that is very low in calories, rich in fiber and potassium, magnesium and low in sugar. For a constipated baby, soak the prunes in water overnight, and serve a teaspoon either with the food, or with the water, or even just as a little dessert. For children with a tendency to be constipated I would always prune on the table, as in many households we can find candies permanently available. I would add them to my baking, to fruit salads, and even to Tofu when baking it as "stuffed turkey" for Christmas for those who think that a meal does not need to be killed for us to celebrate.

12. ***Bee Pollen-*** Can be used only if you know that your child is not allergic to pollen. It is easy to check if your child is allergic to bee pollen by first letting him or her smell it, and then add just one or two little balls of the bee pollen to the food. If there is an allergic reaction, it will show right away. Children that are allergic need to be treated for the kidneys, intestines, and liver. As already mentioned before the rule of thumb is what to eliminate from the diet is more important, rather than adding. For example, I would first start to eliminate meat and dairy. I would never think of medications. If you are allergic, it is a good time to treat the allergy in a natural way. Allergies are not a disease that should be addressed with allergy suppressants, but through stimulation of the immune system and removal of the irritant. However, if your child is not allergic, bee pollen is a significant nutrition addition that enhances the hormonal efficiency of the child as well as a very rich source of plant protein and enzymes. Yes, little children also have active hormones. Not the sexual hormones but many other hormones. By helping with the bee pollen, the immune system will get a healthy smooth and uplifting stimulation, and a very good and healthy source of protein.

Giggling Dr. Green

13. ***Propolis*** -Propolis, also called "bee glue," is a resinous substance that bees use to construct and maintain their hives; it also protects the hive from invading insects.

That product is made by the bee from tree sap for the very natural purpose of self-protection. This way, propolis has been in use in many different health products to restore the immune system efficiency. In Israel, propolis is in use for bedsores and for burn victim's injuries, in hospitals. It helps to heal leaving almost no scars left. Propolis is good for prevention and when sick, additional support for recuperation and strengthening.

14. ***Black Coffee-*** Although coffee is considered to be an unhealthy product in general as we know it, (which is proven to be wrong. The only unhealthy coffee is the coffee with any additives like sugar and milk) if overused. It can actually be healthy if used wisely and in the proper amount, rather than drinking it 8 to 10 times daily and allowing the body to become dependent on it. The black coffee stimulants should not be overlooked, especially in young children's health. After all, when you look carefully through the medication's ingredients, you will often find ingredients that act like coffee as a simulate agent. I would have black coffee in my little Alternative Home Pharmacy for a few reasons, such as when a child is too wide-awake and can not fall asleep or calm down; Just smelling the black coffee for one second or two. It works like a Homeopathic remedy, to calm the child down.

The best six doctors anywhere,
And no one can deny it,
Are sunshine, water, rest, and air,
Exercise and diet.

These six will gladly you attend,
If only you are willing,
your mind they will ease,
your will they will mend,
and charge you not a shilling.

Old Nursery Rhyme

Homeopathy doesn't always work by the obvious rules

It is always advisable to seek advice from a well trained and experienced homeopath if you know one you trust. However, there are times when we need an

152

immediate answer and cannot wait for an appointment. You can find the answer even if you are unprepared for the entire Homeopathy studies.

In my many years of homeopathy experience I conclude; that true Homeopathy is actually based on quantum physics; it has the potential to heal, it is energy based and responds amazingly to the law of synchronicity. On countless occasions, when I was not completely clear what the right remedy should be, I would be amazed how the right remedy would "help me" to be chosen by simple signals. For example, when someone would say - you are always busy as a bee, and my illness called for Apis. Even if I didn't know what to choose for myself - the answer was right there. Or when Debbie suffered chest pain, telling me a dream got me the correct remedy for her.

Sometimes in the midst of my debate of what would be the better choice, my hand would grab the remedy I contemplated, and when I tried to find the one I thought should be better, my hand repeatedly picked the same one up. Not what I wanted, but it worked.

Of course, I do not suggest that Homeopathy is pulling the bunny out of the hat every time. Most of my decisions are based upon my extensive experience and knowledge. Those rare occasions when I was not sure what the best choice would be, I allowed the law of synchronicity and a still, quiet voice to guide my hand. I don't suggest this approach without the wisdom, knowledge, experience and ability to completely clear the mind of outside influences I am blessed to possess. Meaning - let go of my ego and allow universal knowledge to enlighten me. However, there are very good ways, and from my understanding, reliable ways to choose the right remedy even if we don't know and never studied homeopathy. I refer to muscle testing or kinesiology.

For a small child it is possible by just putting the potential remedy on his back or belly and playfully makes him push your hand. If it has weak resistance, it's the wrong remedy.

The right remedy resonates within a child's body energy. However if it is not the right remedy it will not resonate with the body's energy. Since homeopathy is based upon the law of healing similar to similar, a similar resonance will be the correct choice to help the child. I know it sounds as if it is too simplified, but see how simple nature's messages are, how your child will get better and how the message your child sends to you is more accurate than any sophisticated modern medicine machine, lab or test.

Trust yourself; train yourself to rely on your intuition. After all, as long as history has been recorded, intuition has always been acknowledged, appreciated and admired, more than any book knowledge, when it comes to healing. In ancient cultures intuition was considered to be God's word and inspiration, or, divine wisdom. Today, scientists think so highly of learned knowledge assets, that many of us believe there is almost no, or even only very little room for intuition. Let us keep in mind how we are a huge bundle of energy fields, like anything else in the universe, and we are capable of receiving messages without words or voice; without books and computers. It is after all a message the body sends to communicate where it hurts. No two cases are ever exactly alike. Messages are not measurable and cannot be weighed. We are capable of receiving messages that come to us out of nowhere or, without any tools and instruments. The body "talks" and we listen. In addition more than coincidentally, they are the absolute correct messages. In order for that to be true we must silence our ego, because the ego is afraid and is insisting on "knowing" better. Only if we really want to help any fear is just an obstacle. Because the energetic synchronicity functions way better when we do not try too hard to be "smart and know it all".

We allow our ego to get in the way only when we don't trust nature, when we do not trust what we see, smell and feel. Leaving the judgment of what is the best for us or for our child to the universal wisdom, should be our true choice. I strongly believe that the sick child, or adult, sends very clear signals of the troubling condition and the answers are at our disposal. Only when we want to know it all, only when we want to make the decisions and leave them to nothing else but our books- wisdom, we may be caught in the cobwebs of pride, which lures the wisdom to a dead end. I accumulated this wisdom throughout many years of experience. I learned to close my eyes, and allow. Not try to solve the problem, but to attend and allow. Try to listen to all the signals and what they say and you will find those to be the best solution. It works miracles.

Consider, for a moment, this quote from Juvenal, a Roman poet.

"Never does nature say one thing and wisdom another."

Here is a short story as my client's life was saved, I think, only because I gave up my ego, and left the decision to the higher power.

When Shay's young teacher was so sick that she collapsed in class, no one knew what happened to her. The doctors diagnosed her as "Blood vessels grew too small for her blood cells", which really puzzled me. When she came to see me, I was determined to set my wisdom aside, and allow my instincts to guide me, since I truly felt that I had absolutely no clue what her problem was. I opened myself to divine wisdom, and whatever would flow through me I would embrace. (Throughout my career, I felt as though I was just the vessel allowing the universal wisdom flow through me)

The first question I asked her was; do you have allergies? She answered, "Yes, for years I have been taking medications to stop the effects of the allergies".

The answer to this health riddle was spoken into my very soul. The teacher had been overmedicated, by her physician, with far too much antihistamine prescriptions to suppress her allergies. Her problem of which she fainted in class was the lack of blood supply to her legs while standing for a while in class. I explained to her my "thinking", and since she was Shay's biology teacher, it made sense to her. When the medication is supposed to "narrow" the blood vessels in the nose and sinuses, (this is the idea behind allergy medication), the whole body gets that same message. The narrowing of these blood vessels is in order to retard the histamines reaction of the nasal fluids as in response to the allergen. The production of the nasal fluids is the body's way to transport all those "threats" if it stays in the body, and so, some people will respond with diarrhea, some with tearing eyes and runny nose, and some through high fever and profuse sweat. That teacher's reaction to the "invader" was the never stopping runny nose and teary eyes. I would suggest preventing her from certain foods so she can heal her immune system, rather than "forcing "her body to stop the reaction of self preservation and self protection. We would never cover the warning light on our dashboard rather than fixing the problem.

This is what we allow the doctors to do when we allow allergy medications.

Any medication has harmful side effects (no medication heals) and if administered for prolonged time - is deadly. The impact is on the entire being, not just the matter but the mental and emotional realms are eventually harmed as well. Therefore, all vessels in her body tightened up and free blood circulation to the legs, like to the nose blood vessels, was inhibited and delayed.

When the doctors "discovered" that her blood vessels "narrowed so her red blood cells could not flow" nobody made the connection with the prolonged anti allergy, antihistamine prescribed medication. Funny? No, but sad. These damages happen daily to millions of children and adults with allergies, as well as the other "disorders", such as getting prostate problems from high blood pressure medications for adults (now in children as well), men erectile function disorders from diabetes, etc.

Giggling Dr. Green

This lady teacher needed Sulfur 16 LM which would counteract the allergy suppressing medications. The sulfur worked miraculously fast and with astonishing efficiency. The manufactured disease has never occurred since then.

Every time I let go of my ego, I become infinitely more able to observe the true condition of the patient, and then make a decision. This way, I don't jump to conclusions. I do not judge or compare cases, or even decide the right remedy. When we jump into conclusions too fast, we often are not taking the necessary time to truly observe and listen all the way. It happens commonly in our quick fix culture, prescription pad always in hand, doctors have 5 minutes for a patient, and the answer in that ridiculous amount of time is to quiet the symptoms, there is no time to learn what lies behind the complaints. Compare the doctor's prescription writing for every physical complaint to taping shut the mouth of a crying child. "Very good", thinks the doctor, "I have cured the child from crying." A rather ludicrous example, I admit, but a good illustration of my point, I believe. However, if we understand that it is not in the person's long term best interest to simply place a pretty bandage over a gaping wound, we are then able to realize that allowing the body to signal and display its suffering, and support it to complete, naturally, the healing process. Because, once the body has completed the healing process, it has "learned" to deal with the problem, so for the next time, if the same ailment begins to occur, the disease will be simple and easily overcome. As with other challenges we face in life, and as we ride it through them we get stronger and wiser.

To be too concerned the little boy will fall when first riding his little bike, never let go of the two-wheel bike. Their child is so anxious to learn to ride alone as we anxiously hold on and run along. This overprotected child will never learn to keep her/ his balance with the parent holding the back of the bike. When our body is fighting an illness, it is very much the same. The prescription medication makes us feel protected for a time, but then someday we realize how we have never allowed our body to do what it was created to do, and that is to heal and protect itself. Maintain a healthy balance, in mind, body and spirit. If the body is not allowed the tools and time to fight the disease all the way to completion by repeatedly being stopped, it will get the same disease time and time again. If we suppress the body in its effort to overcome - illness, if we work against the body instead of with it - it will never really heal. It may not get the same symptoms again, because the body may express the same illness in a different way, however there will be no lasting health. Like suppressed allergies that turn into asthma, or psoriasis, the body will persist in its efforts to receive the support it requires to enable self-healing.

Giggling Dr. Green

Try to understand how homeopathy works, and if you feel that you cannot make a decision, call your homeopath. Yet, if the latter is unavailable, take the leap of faith, do not think too much and just ask the universe for guidance. Try muscle testing or with the pendulum. You will apply the right remedy. In addition, since you cannot harm with the highly diluted remedies, you can only win. For example, if the nose and eyes are running like a water faucet and you do not find the answer, just stop and think. Does it look as though that person peeled and cut an onion? Well, then it needs to have simply a homeopathic remedy that is made of onion and that would be - Allium Cepa. Even if you just take a real onion and hold it in your hands and very lightly tap along the child's back up and down, it will work like a homeopathic remedy. Homeopathy is simple providing we do not try to understand and control every situation. If we look at the whole picture, choose a remedy that is similar to the symptom, and consider the way it would affect the person had it been given in a bigger amount. Unlike many medications, homeopathy asks you only to watch for the "doesn't make sense" symptoms, and give the same. Never give a remedy against a disease or disorder.

We never know for sure whether our choice was the perfect choice, even after 40 years of seeing it all. Only the results will tell. Because - homeopathy is based upon the quantum physics concept.

You will not find even one respectful and serious homeopathy book, in which the author can give a definite recommended remedy in every given case. My most wonderful homeopathy teacher and mentor from Germany wrote the best and the most detailed Homeopathy books. Even he, a professor for homeopathy in the university in Munich, more than once said to me; "Kido, every healing is an art, and we simply must learn as much as we can, yet, we have to leave the final decision to divine wisdom, since every dis-ease has it's karma". I was very surprised to hear him say that. I was so sure that he would know everything, and that he would never doubt his decisions - but I was wrong. Like every well-trained, knowledgeable homeopath, he also had his doubts. Notice how not two homeopaths will prescribe the same remedy for the same problem. What does that tell us? That the homeopathy does not heal diseases, but heals the person and that each person is a whole world of itself. No two people are alike in any way. The most important difference between homeopathy and the mainstream medication is: we can never harm.

During my studies in Germany, I suffered from ulcerative colitis with Crohn's disease and was in critical condition. My admired mentor could not help me and I was deeply disappointed in my guru. Years later, when I healed (needless to mention; without medication and of course, no surgery), I understood his position much better. In order to heal completely, the homeopathic remedy alone will not be sufficient. Many times, we will have to make major changes in other parts of the sick person's life, whether it is the diet, the environment, or maybe the stress level. In order to choose the right homeopathy, all we really need to do is observe and listen to the story the body or person tells us. With the support and aid in the healing process, never suppress or stop the process. My point is; if you feel you understand the concept behind homeopathy try it. If you are not sure, or too concerned, call a homeopath you trust. I would highly recommend first of all calming down and keeping your child far from medications. Start by applying the harmless, soothing, supporting and strengthening natural means. Only if they do not work and you feel in your heart that you need a mainstream doctor, then do go with your heart. Later, you can resume the natural way, when your child is out of the critical condition.

The more daring among us, understand that these critical moments quickly pass. Those parents dare to continue with reflexology, homeopathy, natural teas etc. Some symptoms are dangerous, however, and need quick and professional assistance. You are not a failure raising your child in the natural way and when absolutely necessary, take your child to a doctor, or emergency room. I myself never took my children to the hospital and succeeded to manage with simple natural applications. Each case must be considered individually and every parent knows his child's limits and strengths best. Healing is a very delicate combination of knowledge, intuition, art and experience, regardless which discipline we choose. There are more intuitive doctors whose rate of misdiagnosing and wrong medicine choice is very low, and there are those, who have to search more and miss more often the right diagnosis and the right application. The same is happening with naturopathic practitioners. If we do not diagnose and just listen to the body needs, disregarding any correct label - can we truly help and heal... The labeling is the biggest thorn on the healing path. The difference; all medications have detrimental, damaging, and even life threatening side effects and worse, if prescribed or administered incorrectly. All surgeries are a total assault on the body. The natural applications have no harmful side effects. The way I would choose, of course, would always be the natural way first, and only if it doesn't solve the problem soon enough or, when there is a life threatening condition, would I resort to the mainstream medicine. I suggest that parents do their best to prevent and learn about the different ways they can help their children before they get sick.

The holistic view

The most important rule in my opinion would be, no matter what the situation or the name of the disease may be, if the physician or practitioner does not see the whole person, they will probably fail in their effort to help. Please do not be shy and timid when at any therapy, and it is your responsibility to draw the practitioner's attention to the whole child. Do not accept when the stomach, foot, nose or any other part with obvious symptoms displayed is addressed.

This is the most vital key for success in any sort of therapy, medicine and healing. The examples I had given in this book about tonsillitis and warts are just examples of a few cases that, without addressing the wholeness, we were doomed to fail in healing.

I remember a 9 year old boy who was such a good student, when suddenly his grades dropped and he could not even write properly any more. The doctor suggested Ritalin. When I saw him I asked about vaccinations or medications he had lately received. I learned that just a few months ago he fell from his horse and was given tetanus shots. That was my clue. I gave him Thuja 16LM to undo the vaccination side effects, and he was fine the next day. No tremors or writing problems any more.

Therefore, here is a little guide for some of the listed homeopathic remedies and what would be the right choice. Remember, it is not written in stone. If one has not completed the task, reevaluate from the start. When you believe you have considered everything, go back slowly, and discover the small information you thought to be unimportant. That may be the very thing that holds the key to unlock the door to your child's health. Try to stay as calm as possible, and know that no matter what, you cannot harm your child with the wrong choice of homeopathy. If it was not the right choice, it just did not do anything. If there is a reaction, just wait until it changes again.

The golden rule is: you can never give too little homeopathy. Only giving too much, provided it is the perfect choice- can create a short term, uncomfortable reaction. Yet, too little will always work when the remedy of choice is the right one for the child.

No two people, even if the labeled disease is the same, will respond exactly the same to the same remedy. So it is important to wait after administering the remedy, and not hurry to repeat it. It is like helping an old woman down the stairs, and if she starts to take a small step on her own we still give her a push. The body received the message and needs no reminder.

Giggling Dr. Green

For example, if you have symptoms like flu, it may mean for you; high fever, perspiring profusely and every joint in your body hurts. You may have an aversion to cooked food, and have no thirst. That would call for a different homeopathic remedy than the same flu in your friend's case, when he is experiencing a low-grade fever, big appetite, shivers and profound thirst. This is a perfect example why the remedies are so different in nature and the reason for so many well-trained homeopaths' errors to choose the correct remedy at first try. My point is; stay away from the diagnosis label. Do not feel inadequate, just look at the signs the person, or your child displays, and go only by them. If we start from the name of the disease, we are sentenced to fail with the choice of remedy! Pay attention to the symptoms, and ignore their common name.

To summarize rule number 1 – get a clear picture of what the child displays that is different from its normal. Do not forget the most important – disposition and unspoken signs, such as redness of the face, body odor, urine odor, cuddliness or restlessness etc.

2. *Homeopathic remedies specifics*

In the effort to understand the Homeopathic remedies, try to remember just one or two very specific modalities of the particular remedy.

Homeopathy in case of Emergency

Helpful key words

Sudden, very red, hot that stays in your hand/**Bell** 16 LM

Nausea, over indulging, competitive/ **Nux -V** 16 LM

Cuts and bruises, burns, assault/ **Arn** 16 LM

 Surgery frostbites (When severe every 2 hours) Cuts and bruises

Ledum 16 LM like Arn 16LM

Old man, pale blue, poisoning /**Ars-A** 16 LM

 Unclean, sewer, filth, bad odor, rotten eggs/ **Sulfur** 16LM

Too. too much of anything / **Rhus- Tox** 16LM

Lack of oxygen, weak, humid damp environment/ **Carbo-V** 16LM

Vaccines, warts, /**Thuja** 16LM

First fever start salty perspiration/ **Ac-P**

Giggling Dr. Green

Clingy, sweet, kind, sensitive, vaccines/ **Puls** 6LM

Rebellious, anti, restless, inflammation/**Cham** 6X

Bee, like bee/Apis 6LM Winy, art, crying gets worse, ball/ **Ign** 6LM

Chapter Seven

Children Cancer

Daniel's parents were both respected medical professionals. Her father was Chief of Staff in a very well known hospital in Israel, and her mother was a pediatric nurse. When the father called me about their 9 years old, he told me his very alarming story. Daniel had been complaining for a few months about hip pain. (Does that explain my alarm when Shay complained about his pain in the hips?) "I didn't take it very seriously, and supposed it was just growing pain. All I gave her was just a few aspirin to calm her pain down and in case there was a little local inflammation." He said. "However, the pain only got worse. Finally, my wife and I decided to have her examined to learn the reason for her pain. Yael, it is the most devastating news we have ever received in our entire lives. We learned that our precious daughter had bone cancer in her hip". He took several deep breaths before he could continue and then he asked, "I have heard so much about you, please, will you see our daughter and can you help her?" I did not hesitate to answer; Of course I will see your daughter, and yes, I believe and hope that I can help her. The same day, they brought Daniel to my office, which, in reality, is not an official office. Since my role model was my grandmother's cousin, I work out of my home office, simple, inviting and not at all pretentious. That was a little strange to them, considering the impression they had from the stories about me. I believe that healing is a form of art and every time I had tried to work in a conventional and impressive office, I felt uninspired and out of place.

We talked about the plan for Daniel. The parent's determination and courage to step outside their professional comfort zone, to consult with a natural health practitioner like myself, was impressive. Without an expensive decorated office, no white coat, no prescription medications, and no x-ray machine - just a simple home office filled with good energy and experience.

I stressed my point of view regarding cancer and explained it to be the last alarm the body sends out to draw our attention to the failing self-defense mechanism. Illustrating verbally how, cutting out and "killing the cancer" is like hitting a crying child to help him calm down. What the body really needs is attention, gentleness, support, different patterns of thinking, a change of diet, and a change of the conditions and circumstances that brought it to the point of cancer. Holding the child while listening to the reason she/he is crying will help the child. Just as listening to the body would help it regain its natural ability to control the protein production and healthy cell multiplication to resume good health.

Cancer is the body's own production, and by no means an evil enemy that comes from outside to invade our cells. Many times in children develop cancer after being overly medicated for any little problem and to suppress infections, rashes, etc. Their self defense mechanism collapsed. Cancer can also appear in children who need to express themselves, when life is substantially different than they would like it to be. For example, when I was a child, friends of my parents immigrated to a different country to their daughter's who were about my age, to great dismay. She had to leave her grandparents, her school and friends, and the only home she had ever known behind and move to a cold, strange country, where she would have no friends or extended family. She was devastated; however, she had no choice. The poor, depressed child died of cancer one year after they moved.

Captivated wildlife often develop cancer the same way. If we listen to the child's emotional pain and worries, especially to the very well behaved child, the pleaser, the sensitive one, the excellent student and the child who would always do beyond any expectation. This child may harbor thoughts, disappointments or worries in order not to hurt his parents or cause any problems. Cancer becomes the only way to express desperation. So we need to be attentive to their emotions. Often parents push their children to be the best in school, star player on the team and perfect in their behavior, look the best, be the best, make their parents be proud of them.

What heavy burdens we place on our child for our personal fulfillment through his or her achievements. Some of these belabored children will withdraw and simply give up the endless pursuit of perfection. However, they cannot just say, "I give up, Mommy. I can't be perfect anymore, Daddy", so instead their bodies cry out with repetitive sinus infections, tonsillitis, or asthma. The list of possible illnesses we may display in protest to stress is very long. When these illnesses begin to show up, we parents see ourselves as best parents (if we push our children to be the best, we need to be the best as well), we will get our child to the doctor and obtain the correct prescription to get rid of the disease, as quickly as possible.

My grandchildren already know that even with a serious illness such as pneumonia my first question would be; what is upsetting you so bad? Or; what is it that you really fear, yet feel obligated to do? My choice of homeopathic remedy and support will always first address the emotions and then the physical complaints. This is my approach to all named cancer as well. I emphasize 'all cancer' because there is no difference what kind of cancer it is. The many different names for cancer are just an artificial invention of the doctors. Cancer can develop anywhere in the body and will point toward the source of the real, buried problem. For example, throat cancer may indicate a speech issue, unacknowledged grief, fear of expressing oneself, painful shyness, or suppressed anger. True physical healing goes all the way to the often hidden emotional distress.

My suggestions for Daniel's recovery were very simple and clear. Not necessarily easy for these representatives of the mainstream to accept, understand and follow, but they received my directives very well. They answered my plan to enable their daughter's body to heal itself with, "Our beautiful Daniel has been given just a few more weeks to live. We'll do anything to help her." I could not promise anything but my experience and trust in nature's power was such that if we obey nature's rules the chances to recover are great.

We completely changed Daniel's diet. She was to receive no dairy, gluten, meat and nothing processed, not even eggs. I began to apply reflexology twice a week and added homeopathy remedies.

Mary was on the line insisting she must come and see me right away, after the first 2 weeks and said that she would not mind coming to a "Doctor's visit" in the doctor's bedroom, because I was down sick myself. We thought it was funny and I agreed to see her, even in my bed. Mary stormed in like a tornado, anxious to share her news. She was holding a file in her hands and shaking like a leaf so much I have to admit, it frightened me. Then she reached out, not caring about my cold, gave me a bear hug and said, "Yael, we just got the newest results for Daniel. There were 3 big tumors, now 2 are completely gone and the third one is just 40% of its size. Do you realize that we can keep Daniel? She is not going to die! All we need is to just continue what we have been doing and she will get better!" Overwhelmed with emotion, we both sat on my bed and cried with joy and relief.

When I moved from Israel to America, I continued to receive updates on Daniel through a mutual family friend. Sadly, at some point Daniel fell away from the healthy lifestyle I suggested to her and passed away when she was only 19 years old. Had I stayed in Israel, and kept her under my healing wings, perhaps she would still be alive, but I cannot say this with any certainty. The patient is either her /his own best friend, or her/his own worst enemy, and in the art of healing all we can do is paint the path, we cannot insist you follow it.

How the Mega force failed Linda

As I was called late at night I could hear the fear in her voice she could not hide. A diagnosis of leukemia for her 12 years old daughter, Linda, provoked this fear. She asked me to help and said she really felt strongly that Linda could overcome it, in a non-invasive way. I met with my friend, Rosie and her husband, Linda's father. My way has always been, restoration of the Immune System, and Linda's mother agreed.

The father, however, was against my natural ways and soon he admitted Linda to the children's hospital in Denver, Colorado where the pediatrician told her parents, "Linda has a very complicated case of Leukemia, and we have to double her chemotherapy. Her chances of survival are only 50%". Need I explain my sorrow on the child's behalf?

Rosie asked me to try to remedy the strong effects of the chemotherapy, but I knew I could not do much for the poor girl. The medications are excessively strong and devastating to the immune system. However, I agreed to try and for that to be possible, I was asked to meet with the treating doctor. When I entered her office she asked me, "What is Homeopathy? Will it undo the chemotherapy? Why would you choose homeopathy?"

Since I liked Linda very much, I cannot deny emotional involvement and replied; "How many children survive your chemotherapy?" The doctor answered; "Well, the truth is that none do. They don't die of cancer, when they die it is always because their body has no resistance left anymore, and they succumb to pneumonia or any other simple virus." So, why would you double the dose for Linda? I asked. I was very angry at the system already when she replied, "We have to go by the books. The books are ancient and the hospital has not changed anything in the procedure for treating cancer in ages. Quite the contrary; in fact the chemotherapy has only gotten deadlier."

Well, I said, Homeopathy works by healing 'similar with similar'. In Linda's case, the homeopathy would remind her body how to deal with the cause for her symptoms that brought to your diagnosis and grim prognosis. I would never fight the cancer cells; there is a reason for her young body to have created them in the first place. Therefore instead of fighting the cancerous cells, I will restore Linda's ability to heal her own body. The reason for the cancer needs to be addressed so she could live.

Giggling Dr. Green

My eyes filled with tears as I answered her earlier question; No, homeopathic remedies cannot counteract your deadly chemotherapy, unfortunately. But as for you- how can you look in the mirror each morning?

I admit having no mercy for that pediatrician with my parting comment. She was just doing her job the best she could, but watching so many children die in vain, will she ever ask herself , "Why"? And insist on change?

Linda received the double potent chemotherapy treatments. The law is on the side of MEGA Force and its feigned ignorance. Parents face the danger of being prosecuted for choosing not to use the mainstream medical path and having their children taken away from them. This is truly my biggest nightmare, reminding me so much of the Inquisition era in Spain, burning people at the stake for thinking differently than the church permitted. Communist regimes still execute people who express different opinions than the government mandates as truth. If the government assumes the right to punish the parents who choose to help their children in different ways than what the mainstream medical field offers, the government should be aware and comply with advanced studies, research and knowledge. Every independent, scientific study in the past 75 years has concluded with one foundational truth: *Strengthening the immune system is the correct and sole treatment for cancer*. Continuing to impose wrong and harmful treatments on all these innocent children and simply kill them in the name of 'medicine' is the biggest crime of our century. It is the MEGA Force and economically involved industries that lead to these monstrous rules. The precious lives of our children are not behind their drive and purpose. If mainstream medicine had no lobbyist in Congress and cancer would be treated naturally, the economy in America would be devastated. As Al Carter the author of "The cancer answer" said so poignantly, "More people live off cancer, than die from it". This is the end to Linda's story; she passed away about one month after admission to the hospital. During that final month, she suffered so much pain, as they subjected her to one surgery after another. Those surgeries were supposed to correct the side effects of the chemotherapy treatments. How ironic?

In her diary she wrote about her dream to return to her home country. Yet, her parents could not make that dream come true. She wrote how she knew she would pass away at the age of 12, and described the way she would like to be dressed for her funeral.

In her medical history there were many bouts with tonsillitis, all treated with courses of antibiotics, prior to her leukemia diagnosis. Looking back, I wonder what the chemotherapy was to cure. Did it help Linda to express her sadness and homesickness? Did all the surgeries help her to address the deep despair in her soul? No, of course not, they just cut out the result of her sadness and despair, put a band-aid over the deeper emotional wounds, and sent her off to her funeral. Linda's story represents countless other similar stories, children forced by governmental rules and regulations as well as the MEGA Force, to receive the dreaded chemo, and then prepare to

Chapter Eight

Wake up and save our children

I deeply regret the need to write these facts which are so well known, and yet ignored. I call all of you parents to open your eyes and join the fight against this legitimate, wholesale slaughter of our children.

As a child, I was always puzzled by cancer. That is odd to say, I know, why should cancer trouble a child? Childhood should be fun and carefree. I am not certain why, but I was always a very curious child, and cancer seemed to be a puzzle to solve. Perhaps it was a sense of mission driving me? After all, I grew up to study cancer as a near-obsession, reading case studies from all over the world, exploring different schools of thought, different approaches and strategies. In more than 43 years of practicing the healing arts, I had countless opportunities to help cancer diagnosed people- heal themselves. I would never deny that this radically different approach flies in the face of mainstream medicine.

To this day friends and patients thank God for taking my advice, as intuitive or even crazy as it seemed at times. Consultations and anger management are vitally important in cancer treatments.

As I continue my research into alternative methods of - not fighting but understanding dis-ease, the more I find my theories are confirmed and liable. My views on my approach to curing cancer only grow stronger by the year. There is a debate within alternative health circles on whether the MEGA Force does its harm knowingly or not. Does the vast complex of pharmaceutical companies and doctors who do their bidding, truly and honestly believe it has the best approach to cancer? Does mainstream medicine really believe that pumping patients full of cell-destroying drugs is the right way? Does mainstream medicine truly believe that the burning of cells may heal the patient of cancer? On the other hand, does mainstream medicine knowingly destroy lives in the quest for a fatter bottom line? Perhaps I am a little cynical, but after years in the "trenches" of medicine as it were, I tend to believe the latter. Nevertheless, this is my personal opinion. Still, you cannot blame me for asking the question, as perhaps you have as well. How expensive are all those mainstream treatments of cancer? The pills, the many I.V. drips, and the chemicals patients must take to battle the side effects of the original treatments? Not even the most pure-hearted doctor would deny that this is a highly profitable operation. Why put all that profit at risk?

It is an absurd thought. It took me more than 60 years to wake up from my illusions. Some people are more realistic, and wake up much sooner in their lives. However, bear with me for a moment. Just think of that profit-making machinery in place. It is like a business plan and product line that has worked for so long. The chemotherapy, the radiation, the MRI machines, syringes, health insurance, special treatments, social workers, nurses, hospice, breast reconstructions, wigs, surgery rooms and equipment, the dizzying network of products and services that cancer patients require. They all create a huge, fearsome industry around a very dreadful yet very cost-effective disease. If the system is making such wealth this way, why change the approach? The entire economy would tumble down like a card house and the fraud as it is would be exposed.

The approach of all of us natural health practitioners and doctors, who have been following ancient paths to health, is way simpler, sensible and humble. When I think of battling cancer I think; juicers, reflexology treatments, guided visualization, homeopathy, PEMF therapy and consultations, Yoga, anger-management, healthy diet, relaxation, acupuncture, Chinese herbs, Tai chi, exposure to natural environment, halting any and all medications, aroma therapy, Bach flowers, light therapy, chiropractic and so many more possible ways. They are significantly less expensive, easy to understand, non-invasive, non toxic or harmful. True, nobody gets rich off it. I hesitate to write this, but this is the only true reason for the MEGA Force to continue knowingly without any ethical morals and respect to life rather than money -to treat cancer sufferers with their old, useless, devastating, deadly methods.

Thus, only those who have the courage to shake off these dangerous medical-establishment brain-washing from their heads, only those who understand the reasoning behind the ancient theories, that had helped for centuries millions of people, have a better chance of surviving cancer. Better chance than through the mainstream treatments - a given truth. There is no legal justification or moral reason why the AMA and FDA threaten to strip practitioners of alternative methods of their licenses or even arrest them for "practicing medicine without a license." The only motive behind it is not the true best of the citizens, but their own monetary benefits.

Giggling Dr. Green

Think about it in terms of numbers. Consider the statistics. How many people die of cancer every year, after a long horrendous painful and desperate struggle? If such astronomical sums of money are poured into cancer research, why has it not been eradicated? There is so much research conducted for the past decades in this cancer, so, where is all this knowledge going? Why is the mainstream "medicine" still circling around the same approach if the results are nothing but more medications, more machinery, more computerized equipment, more suffering, and ultimately more painful untimely deaths? Which science other than cancer required these vast amounts of dollars, hours, staff, labs, poor Guinea pigs, mice, rats, and even people volunteering to test the "new" miraculous medications for the final answer to cancer? Thus the truth is that the answer is hidden from us and will never even appear on the horizon? Will it ever? Have they ever considered that it is not, in fact, a disease, but a failure, a bankruptcy of the immune system? Moreover, if that is the case, what of the MEGA Force's approach of chemically attacking that immune system even more? Why doesn't the medical establishment alter its angle of attack, and instead of killing the body (by killing the cells, because the body's cells), help people to rebuild and recover their broken down immune system? Let us suppose, just for the sake of argument, that the medical establishment deserved a monopoly on treating cancer that its methods for "healing" cancer represented the best true medical science could offer. Why is the cancer mortality rate still skyrocketing?

Instead, the complementary medicine approach which enhances the autoimmune system, restores the balance of the body, mind and soul needs, are considered to be outlawed, so only the "real doctors" would have the access to these natural healing means? What do mainstream doctors know about health? Balance? Restoration of the autoimmune system? The wholeness of body, mind and spirit? The need to help the sick person to restore that balance of his or her being? Did you ever hear about any chemotherapy medication that helps to heal depression? (one of the known triggers for cancer), certainly not, but research shows the devastating number of chemotherapy patients who are struggling with depression, and those who even commit suicide, simply to be done with the barbaric treatments, even more than the suffer of cancer itself. Does radiation aid in the healing grief? Is there any mastectomy that heals divorce trauma? Is there any surgery that could help a child to overcome the trauma of loss of a close family member? Is there any chemotherapy ingredient that heals negligence or abuse? When will the medicine be so honest and truthful to admit that these may be the main possible reasons for all the devastating diseases? Addressing the reason for the illness evidently is the only way that can truly help the individual restore good and sustaining health.

Who has not heard the magic bullet of: "If in 5 years there is no relapse…"? Real healing will not need 5 years for the ominous, almost sure relapse, because the very true healing is about subsiding the cause of the disease and helping the child or adult learn how to approach a different path to health and maintain that beautiful health. Physically, mentally and emotionally versus by cutting out body parts, (which makes depression even worse), but by helping the child deal and manage his sadness, fear or any other negative emotions, accompanied with a nice healthy change in his or her diet and grow to be healthy and vibrant. This is true health. No relapses on anyone's agenda but getting better each day. This is what true health care, medicine and the responsibility of the FDA and AMA should be. This is what they were elected for, this is what they are paid for, and this is what they swore to offer you, me and our children for as long as they serve. Please, pray with me that a day will come in the world of mainstream healthcare where high values, integrity, and the entire patient's well-being are deemed more important than the profit margin.

It leads to other questions that make one wonder about the complicity of other organizations. For instance, if the FDA were actually concerned about the public's health, why doesn't it shut down the fast-food industry with its heart-killing hamburgers and fried chicken? The colorful candies and addictive beverages? Why doesn't it ban junk food, or even imported food from China, a country with a food industry that even puts melanin in baby food? Why does the FDA give the nod to harmful, addictive and even mutilating medications for babies, and forcefully prohibit the harmless healing treatments of alternative medicine? Why does the FDA still sanction, in fact promote, the dreadful, horrific treatments for cancer-suffers, knowing it is in fact speeding these victims' path to death, callously turning its back on its commitment to promote health and save lives? The MEGA Force represents one of biggest corruptions in history, and yet they maintain control over our health and our children's health.

Our ignorance makes us complacent in this. So many of us believe what the media tells us; we do not check out their assertions, we do not question their agendas, we do not even ask simple common-sense questions. And when we do, it is often too late -when, already sick, our loved ones or we have realized the con job that has been pulled on us by the MEGA Force. Even if you do ask the doctor, he or she would stare at how you dare doubt their seniority and authority over our health.

Giggling Dr. Green

Thus, I want to share with you how I came to find my way past all this medical-establishment brainwashing and see the light about cancer. I have touched on this in other chapters as well, but the fundamentals of my view bear some elaboration.

Cancer is not a Disease

Why do I repeatedly claim that cancer is not a disease? Cancer is not a disease because it does not display any "fighting" symptoms. It is a condition of which the body simply cannot fight any more. Like the child that sits in a corner and does not take part in any activity and just sits there silently, doesn't play, doesn't argue or cry, never smiles, yet, doesn't move away either. This child has so much pain to bear, yet, does not display any signs of discomfort. The child gave up on trying. Every time it would say something that hurt or bothered him or her, it would be silenced by his father, mother or teacher. The child has so much pain inside his little body and seems as if nothing concerns him anymore, from the outside. Until, one day the catastrophe hits and this child commits a terrible act. This is how Cancer develops. The body displayed many differences of imbalance, discomfort, indigestion of certain foods, unhappiness that could never be expressed, fear, shocking news he could not deal with other than a rash, or sore throat, for a long time. (Other than cancer developed as a vaccine result - which is the worst immune system killer). Yet, for each one of the physical symptoms we wrongfully call disease, he or she was promptly medicated. No fever was "allowed", or diarrhea to happen. When the child cried, he was prompted to stop crying "like a baby". When mom and dad separated, he was hushed from expressing his pain, fear and worry. The person whether child or adult accumulated too many "stoppers" of any physical displays, until it stopped getting sick anymore. Only the "no disease" would definitely alarm me and for a good reason. When a child is "never" sick, it is a sign of being very sick. Very sick; because the body is: "too sick to display sickness". This is the worst situation. This is when the autoimmune system is paralyzed and the cancer cells can thrive. Or, if it is not cancer it can be any other kind of autoimmune disorder or chronic disease. The "real disease" will "cry out" so loud that the body will have to fight. In a chronic stage, on the same list as the different cancers and the "old people disease" belong, the fighting is so dull and so silent, that it resembles the weak and devastated army, or very old woman who cannot fight her attacker. When the body surrenders and gives up like the little child that sits in the corner and is just numb to all his friends and party. This is the reason why I repeatedly say that; cancer is not a disease. It is a bankruptcy of the immune system. It is not caused by a virus or bacteria, fungus or any outside agent the mainstream medicine so eagerly blames. When the hormonal system, which is a crucial part of the immune system, loses control of the cells multiplication. Then the body creates uncontrolled protein chains different from the natural normal protein the body builds when healthy. These cells have no connection and are not steered by the brain and the "general rules and regulations" of the healthy body which makes these protein cells very weak. When the doctors talk about an aggressive cancer, they better say: "very weak immune system". That would much better describe the truth. If we try to kill the cancer cells, we actually cause it to spread even more. It is like an inflammation or boil. Or, let's take appendicitis for example. This condition turns to be life threatening only when the appendix ruptures and the whole inner abdomen is filled with the pus. However, as long as it stays closed, the pus will be contained in the appendix until the inflammation will subside. (It is just a metaphor for the concentration in one tumor or cyst. I do not suggest avoiding surgery if needed in appendicitis case) the "fight" against the cancer cells is pretty similar. As long as the body contains the cancer cells in the tumor, these cells will not spread all over the body through the bloodstream and lymphatic paths. Once the cancer tumor is cut, the cancer cells will be transported by the blood through the entire body. With every injury, the most important function of the self healing mechanism is to rush blood serum and lymphatic fluid to the injury in order to "repair" and "close" the wound. That means the body will need more cells to regenerate the injured tissue. The same happens also when the tumor is surgically removed and the body thrives to heal and repair the damaged organ and tissue. This is when the surgery actually stimulates cell metastasizing in a higher demand than was needed before the surgery. Yet, the multiplication system of the body has been already compromised and distorted, so, now, it is losing even more control; the test will say; the cancer metastasized.

I am not surprised every time I hear that "the cancer returned". The truth is not that the cancer returned but that the body succumbed to the cheating. The truth is; the cancer was never removed because and has never been healed. Thus, the reason for the cancerous disorder has never been addressed. In order to heal the cancer should never be removed. The only thing that should be removed is; the reason for the cancer! All that happens by removing cancer is nothing but a deeper problem and complication of the situation. By removing the tumor, the body will not stop the cells "wild multiplication" as the tumor will only create new tumors in different parts of the body. The child will be just more disappointed, sadder and will feel lonelier and not understood. On top of its original suffering now the child has to struggle with pain, hospitalization, isolation, fear, facing death, enduring the most horrible side effects of the chemotherapy, medications, surgery and a mutilated distorted body. The child will now "join" a new group of children and see his own reflection when looking at them. He will see how his condition is getting his whole family together at his or her bedside and make him or her think, if that could be a way to "recover" at least his family if not himself. That trauma is unforgettable for life, on top of the entire traumatic path leading to his gloomy present. But, if you strengthen and enhance the immune system, the cancer cells die off and the tumor recedes. We see it every day even in people who have been diagnosed with fourth-stage cancer, and were told by their doctors the dreadful news that they had only a few more weeks to live. The sudden remissions of these so-called "miracle" cases were hardly miracles. They happen through a different yet healthy approach to the immune system, respecting the cause for cancer, by regarding trauma and most importantly cherishing the life force etc. The ability to deal with emotions and life obstacles must always be considered as an immune system as well. It is feasible. Had it not been possible, we would not hear and see numerous cases of recovery without any mainstream medicine intervention. For me, the natural way is the only way. I simply thought and experienced for many years the same scenario. Even on myself, on my own body. Now, doctors have a funny way of explaining these sudden remissions away, often claiming something like; "Well, it was probably not cancer." Alternatively, they have even been known to say; "Sometimes spontaneous healing happens, unrelated to the quackery of alternative medicine." If so, then why not give more people the chance to have that "sometimes" opportunity before starting the killing procedures? Like Dr, Ben-Shahar said to me 25 years ago: "I have been chief of staff here in the Haifa Hospital for 15 years. We know that every patient that comes in on his feet will eventually be carried out covered with the linen sheet. We go by the old books that were written 50 years ago. We over do the amounts and strengthen the chemotherapy medications. We burn people with radiation and poison them with chemotherapy. It is just a matter of time. Yet, deep in my heart I know that it is the wrong way. It is the hospital policy to go by these old books. I know that we should have learned from you and people like you". On the other hand, maybe the recovery was "thanks" to the chemotherapy (which is a turning reason on its head: recovery happens IN SPITE OF chemotherapy). This is the real quackery. These recoveries happened due to the person's strength, his or her inner mental, emotional, and physical inner strength. In other words: the autoimmune system.

Many of you dear readers may think my approach is indeed quackery or witchcraft. I cannot blame your skepticism. I would not like you to blindly believe in the dubious wisdom of the medical establishment, yet on the other hand, I certainly do not want you to blindly believe in me either. I encourage you to look

Giggling Dr. Green

into the vast store of published research, by renowned and respected doctors such as Dr. Candace Pert, Dr. Rosenblum, Dr. McTaggart, Gary Zukav, Dr. Campbell, Dr. Stone, Dr. A.Weil, Dr. Sandmann, Dr. B. Lipton, Dr. Ganot in the Beer-Sheva University, Dr. Gerber, among many others who have undertaken rigorous scientific studies to prove the effectiveness of alternative approach to curing cancer over the 20 to 30 years of intensive exploration. The most shocking are the doctors who were once on the "other side". Those who once believed in conventional cancer treatments and who finally woke up to the eminent truth

Cancer does not just magically appear. We have to look at the chain of events that brings the person to get cancer. Moreover, just as we look at a person's whole history, we must keep our gaze on the person. That is the key: Cancer is a self-made condition, not a disease. Looking for solutions outside the patient is the first step away from the correct path. We need to look inside the patient himself - and into his past as well as in his present. You see, it requires a major chain of events, hocks, traumas and unresolved, unsettling events in a person's life - in order to induce a body to "give up on life." Our bodies usually work like this: our healthy cells multiply to replace dead and regenerate organs, as well as maintain the constant vital activity, like breathing, metabolizing, heartbeat, filtering toxins, think etc.

This routine continues throughout life. This IS, by definition, life. The healthy cells are cells the body produces, simple as that. We constantly regenerate and stay alive. So why would this program suddenly go awry? Why would the body suddenly just go amok? If this system works so well, why would a body simply one day start to produce defective cells that violate the body's normal life-preserving program that has served it so well up to now? Why would a normal, healthy body producing normal, healthy cells, just give up on its normal task in such a situation; destroying these occasional abnormal cells and getting them out of the system? It is a question answered in part by considering the cultures and civilizations of the world: Why do different cultures with different nutrition habits, lifestyles and climates host such healthy people, and have such low cancer rates?

They probably live in synchronicity with nature, as well as good interaction between the cells and the body's functions. Any balance disturbance creates a domino effect -collapse of the system. (The best example for that disturbance would be due to vaccinations/medications).

Look at our own country. Why is the number of children with cancer growing every month, a country that is supposed to be the most advanced in the world, a shining beacon to the rest of humanity? Instead of looking for the answer,

Giggling Dr. Green

we believe what we have been told: "It is because of 1,001 reasons we have no control over."

Do you still believe this foolishness? I don't.

The first shot

Some of these questions answer themselves, but others need to be addressed more directly. Part of the problem goes back to childhood immunizations. Immunizations are a sort of sacred cow of western medicine. Parents feel they must get them for their children or they will surely endanger their health. Of course, all of us want to protect our children and I cannot fault responsible parents. But in this case, good intentions have bad results. Assuming we are doing the best for our children by introducing their systems to a chain of "weakened" viruses and bacteria in order to protect them from illnesses.

The problem is that these weakened bacteria and viruses are hard to fight. They are simply not potent enough to inspire the immune system to "declare war" on the invader. The immune system never rises to challenge because it does not feel it's "worthwhile", and so these immunizations, whether it's inoculated foreign proteins, protein chains, viruses or bacteria - take up residence in the body- forever. They are never fought off or discharged from the body; nor are they integrated into the body's immune system. From that point on- the body has put up with the new "resident" it cannot get rid of nor fight and thus this immunization that was supposed to help, ends up actually hurting the body through deliberately inoculating toxic protein. It is like a splinter you cannot get out, it seems bothersome but small and inconsequential and so after a while you may forget about it. However, the splinter continues doing damage, developing a pocket of pus and subtle inflammation.

As little we know about genetics and why children look like one parent or another, or even may resemble a more distant relative such as an uncle or a grandparent. We know that just as eye color or skin tone may be inherited, so do health problems or even certain health tendencies be inherited from a father or a grandmother. We need only look at someone's family history to get a sense of his health liabilities or tendencies. In official language, doctors often talk about "medical predispositions". Predisposition is nothing more than a genetically inherited tendency to certain sensitivities to condition that if triggered, will manifest a certain disease or disorder. The trick is to avoid the "trigger." Take diabetes for example; a condition that lays dormant and could never flare up unless triggered. The same goes for heart diseases, or neurological diseases etc. and finally, cancer.

My father died of stomach cancer, but it does not necessarily mean I will die of it, too. I have a choice. I can choose to live a different lifestyle than he did, eat a different diet; I can avoid smoking and try to foster a positive healthy attitude. Through choosing to avoid all those triggers, I choose to stay well. This proves that genetics in fact plays a very small part (3%) in the reason why any tendency sometimes blooms into a full-blown disease.

When tendencies in the family stretch way back into the family tree, perhaps even for multiple generations, whether it's pneumonia, paralysis or tuberculosis, for instance, a child can still carry this tendency in his genes and yet live his entire life without ever getting the disease - unless it's triggered. Cancer, arthritis, MS, heart disease, gallbladder, liver and kidney disorders, diabetes, psoriasis and many skin conditions belong to that same category.

We even see many times how in a family all siblings and parties will suffer the same disease, because the same attitudes, the same foods and medicine use are part of their lifestyle. So why would an obese mother not raise obese children and all the family may well develop heart conditions?

When children receive the first immunization shot that is supposed to "help" them, their bodies - sensitive, vulnerable and unprotected - are actually assaulted. That should not come as any surprise. Their bodies just started to build their auto immune systems. And as they go along their body gradually will strengthen that life saving system. The problem is how these immunizations which introduce a weakened virus or bacteria into the children's systems, can act as a trigger. What if one of these inherited tendencies flares up BECAUSE of an immunization? I have seen many children suffer this strange, ironic fate; they were healthy and active up to the point where they got their first shot. Only then did they begin to exhibit strange symptoms.

The concept may be hard for you to accept. Naturally, all parents want the best for their children; between that and adult peer pressure; they feel it is absolutely essential to get the shots for their children. On top the fear of losing their child to the government if this "negligence" of withholding immunization shots is discovered. And when the child does show a reaction to the shot? The doctors easily explain this away as some vague, "normal" reaction and has nothing to do with the shot itself. However, ignoring such a reaction of distress to a shot is very dangerous. Take the case of "Johnny," a case I am very familiar with. After getting his first immunization shot, he displayed alarming obvious symptoms of

Giggling Dr. Green

severe damage to his neurological system; in short, he had a major seizure attack. The "good doctor" went right along with the rest of the battery of shots, ignoring the evidence right before his eyes.

In the previous chapters, I explained through an analogy what happens when the body receives the vaccinations and what actually happens when the child gets them. It would be very interesting to see which parent would dare to take these shots for him or herself as an adult, knowing the danger they are facing. On the other hand, how willing would a doctor be to subject himself or herself to this battery of shots?

In another case, Amira was 13 when she got the mandatory TB shot in school, and shortly afterwards came down with a sore throat. She had received antibiotics and was sent home, with the assurance that it had nothing to do with the shots. After the second round of antibiotics the disaster hit. Amira suffered paralysis in her lower body that stayed with her for the entire life. Tests indicated that Amira had suffered a TB attack in her lower spine. All the steroids and antibiotics she had been given IV did not change anything. She was destined to stay paralyzed for the rest of her life.

On the other hand, Shay was the same age, with the very same lifestyle yet I did not let him get the shot. He is fine. They are both 32 years old. One beautiful princess is in a wheelchair and the other one is dancing.

In 1988, Hadera, Israel was alarmed by a few polio cases that broke out due to the fresh water supply being contaminated by sewage. What was the health department's first response? Enforcing the immediate vaccination of all the children in the city. After the problem had been addressed, some very gruesome facts emerged; the children who had come down with polio had been vaccinated. In that same survey, those that were healthy had not been vaccinated for some reason.

We can see, when the vaccination "hits" the predisposition, the body can react in a very negative way and be harmed forever. When the FDA and physicians are confronted regarding the all-too-obvious complications that come out of the vaccinations, their response is always the same: "Statistically speaking, the percentage of the harmed children is very low". Sad and devastating for two reasons: First, who would agree to put their child among the 10 percent (in reality the percentage is alarming) that would suffer? In addition, the second reason is; it is simply not true. They can still claim the statistical numbers because they deny the correlation between the many complications and the vaccinations. They blame the mercury that preserves the vaccination. The statistics are based upon the number of children vaccinated, yet, does not make the correlation between the vast numbers of ADD, MS, Cancer, Arthritis, SDS, Psoriasis , Liver cirrhosis, Kidney failures, Diabetes and Autism. If I continued on, the list would make this book into a yellow pages book of disease and health disorders.

I argue the idea that the added mercury to preserve the vaccines causes all or most complications arising from vaccines. And what about the Hepatitis in the vaccine bath? Those are unjustified and misleading explanations made up in order to enable the undisrupted mandatory vaccination, a flagrant piece of medical-establishment insanity. If people were to be outraged enough and demand change, the mercury would be taken out, of course, but a different preservative would take its place. Meanwhile, the mortality and complication rate would be the same, if not get even worse. Instead of the "autism epidemic" we would be seeing a "new" neurological disorder epidemic with a new name, new industry thriving off it and "new" misleading explanations. The children and families suffering would stay the same, of course, but with a new name, different symptoms, which will in turn require a new round of madness of the MEGA Force: requiring, of course, new experts, new therapies, new support tools and new medications. In other words, a new surge of prosperity and wealth for the medicine industry. As of now, mainstream medicine is claiming that autism is "A new epidemic." What a false and misleading claim. What we can really chalk up this "new epidemic" to is the government's policy of enforcing vaccinations. Scientists know it, parents with children who have succumbed to this "new epidemic" know it, yet no one is willing to step up and stop this insanity and mass murder. And what of this phrase that is supposed to bring us such comfort, "It is FDA-approved?" How pathetic. Is it truly for the guarantee of our children's health? If anything, this is the best way to guarantee future prosperity for the medical establishment, by destroying the immune systems of all the children born in the USA, and the other very "advanced" countries. Unfortunately, very few are aware that it is their responsibility to - avoid anything that has been approved by the FDA, and choose to take the opposite route for their own health's sake.

It reminds me of that sad joke: A man goes to the doctor. When he comes out with a prescription, he goes to the pharmacy and the pharmacist gives him the medication the doctor prescribed. On his way out of the pharmacy the man tosses the medication into the trash can. His surprised friend asks what he was doing. The man replies, "The doctor wants to live, so he gives me a prescription. The pharmacist wants to live, so he sells me the medicine. I want to live, so I toss it out."

Giggling Dr. Green

A joke? Maybe. Sadly, it is the truth. When the children receive the vaccination, their immune system has been compromised for the rest of their lives. Then what happens to the more than 60 percent of children who have some kind of predisposition? The illnesses start to manifest in the forms of autism, SIDS, liver diseases, kidney disorders, brain disorders, learning disorders, ADD, ADHD, cancer, deformations and much more. This horrible injustice and horrific damage we allow the government to do to our innocent, helpless babies who turn out to be crippled adults, society has to support forever, if they are even lucky enough to grow up in a society that offers such support - is too gruesome to grasp. The poor victims who have to grow up in less fortunate circumstances turn into miserable creatures that once upon a time, were born completely healthy little babies. It was just the establishment of "mandatory" health directors that took away their right to live happy, healthy, self-sufficient, independent and free. I consider this nothing less than a massive cruel crime towards our society.

Vaccination is just one point at which the immune system is "softened up" for the ravages of cancer. For the next step, look no further than your grocery store, where "modern nutrition" is sold for infants. This is another assault on the children's immune system. Any baby food in a sealed container, sitting on a supermarket shelf, is harmful and debilitating food for babies. I might even go so far and call it; sheer poison. Babies were not born to eat anything but mother's milk. Babies were not born to be calves, nor little goats. (Personally I do not know even one bunny mother who would feed her little bunnies with elephant milk.)

Babies were not born with a manual that tells them how to break down the chemical chains of the different powders, pastes, jars and cans offered as "baby food" in supermarkets.

Babies were also not born to eat preserved food with "added vitamins." This is a monstrous invention of the last century, and is just getting worse every day.

The interesting observations we made when we saw American babies when we first arrived was how they all had unusually large heads. It sounds funny, but the underlying truth is serious stuff. It was true of any of the babies who grew up on any kind of baby formula. On the other hand, breastfed babies had a normal size head, much like those we had seen in countries where a mother's convenience is not so heavily catered to in the grocery stores. One famous pediatrician had this to say to a mother who complained that her baby refused to eat baby formula. She told her; "I'm dying to see YOU eat that food. Try it just once and tell me if you would ever open your mouth again to eat it. Do you think babies are stupid?" She

Giggling Dr. Green

made it perfectly clear how she felt about artificial baby food. You see, in mother's milk, the baby gets the most important immune-system ingredients. The mother's milk is the right formula for the baby, whereas cow milk is perfect for a calf. A baby will not stand up within a few minutes after it is born, it will take a good few months to a year. The cow milk is way too heavy for the little liver to digest and the little body cannot utilize it. Let alone the baby's kidneys that have to carry the burden of this strange indigestible fat and protein.

Research has clearly shown that people who grew up on mother's milk had a much healthier and efficient autoimmune system than those who grew up on any other kind of artificial industrial so called "nutrition". Though my opinion is not very popular, I still think the FDA has gone far reaching in damaging the children when approving any other baby food than natural, mother milk, or homemade natural health food. Before Remedia, Similac and Gerber existed; women would actually give their own breast milk to other women who could not nurse their babies. This was the original "baby food." The first year of nutrition, as well as any medication or vaccination, will have the most profound impact on the future health of the baby. This first year is the crucial foundation for the child's future. And faulty nutrition is another factor in compromising or weakening the child's immune system.

Furthermore, this early immune system status can determine the intelligence of the baby. It makes sense; after all, the brain is part of the body. If the kidney, liver, or spleen do not receive the proper nutrition, or are harmed by vaccinations, the immune system has been compromised. The brain development will suffer the consequences as well. Add in the fact that babies must work to nurse at their mother's breast, and the bottle just flows easily. The sucking action is a vital factor in brain development as it trains the sphincters center in the brain, and has a major impact on the whole brain development

Conquer fear with knowledge

Let the baby actually experience and "practice," so to speak, health challenges and learn to overcome them. However, modern lifestyle as well as medical rules and regulations destroy this little human body right to grow strength and resilience. Mothers have to work overtime to "save" their babies from a number of minor ailments, like these widespread myths; "Watch out for fevers they cause convulsions!" "Vomiting causes dehydration and even death!" "Diarrhea may be deadly!" "Ear infection harms the brain and brain development!"

Giggling Dr. Green

"Stop this rash before it spreads!" "A small scratch can turn into tetanus!" This spiral of anxiety can turn the most sensible mother into a ball of fear.

These scare tactics are courtesy of the pharmaceutical companies that claim to have an answer for everything. They profit from scaring poor parents with these dreadful consequences unless the mother and father run out and buy strong medication immediately! Thus, every well-meaning, caring parent searches for the best medicine to immediately stop even the most minor suffering of his or her child as soon as possible. Those who do not reach for some magic syrup or medicine face criticism, ostracism, peer pressure and alienation from friends and family. My daughter had to leave a dinner table at her own Father's house when he blamed and yelled at her for listening to the nonsense ideas of medication free child care. She has always been very courageous when attacked for her health approach. She has three very healthy children who still live medication and vaccination free and overcome every disease just naturally without any "catastrophes" and hospitals,) and maybe even lose their children to the government due to "child neglect." I get the shivers down my back to think of all these parents did was try to help their child develop and strengthen his own immune system to overcome future diseases, to bolster the body to fight off any intruders so that next time, perhaps at a later age the intruder will not have the power to harm it anymore. Is this a crime? Should any parent be punished for claiming the child's right to develop his auto immune system to protect it from all the horrific diseases the children endure these past 20 to 30 years? The irony is: The FDA makes vaccinations mandatory and it's considered to be a crime named-child neglect if parents choose not to dope their kids.

In reality, who are the ruthless criminals here? The answer is; the FDA and MEGA Force. I would never raise my children in such a dictatorial, merciless, corrupt medical regime. All that was mentioned, turns babies even more prone to cancer, and is all solely to enable the medical establishment to cut off the power of their own immune system. I suggest instead, to every parent; try natural avenues before reaching out to any suppressive medication, whether it's a syrup, pill or sugar drop. Even those "innocent" ointments to soothe or stop an itch can damage the immune system.

For instance, if a child repeatedly has tonsillitis, doctors often remove his tonsils; the very signaling system that something is wrong with the child's health is removed! But the body will not be any healthier from now on. The reason for the tonsillitis is not in the tonsils. The better option is to look for the reason for the repeated tonsillitis. Here are some of the possible causes I would search for and address before that invasive, irreversible, harmful and useless procedure: Look for food sensitivity. One of the most common sensitivities of young children, (adults as well), are food products derived from cows, whether it's milk, cheese, yogurt, ice cream, butter, cake, cookies, or any other dairy product.

The other irritant of the tonsils could be teething. Would we pull the teeth out if they were causing the child discomfort? Of course not. By the same token, we should not cut the tonsils out.

Another culprit could be gluten in the baby food. (Gluten is good only for the food industry, not for people). I would look at the neck muscles to see if there is any strained muscle that needs a slight chiropractic adjustment, or maybe a cranial-sacral treatment or reflexology. I would look into changing the way the baby sits in the high chair, stroller, or the way he lays in his crib, or car seat. Some parents believe that a baby's head should be elevated while lying in his crib. I disagree; I think that babies were born to lay straight and flat. That helps to develop a healthy spine, as well as healthy functioning inner organs. When the child is a little older, I would check for the possibility of any kind of unexpressed emotional trauma, or even evidence of molestation. There are many underlying reasons to look for when a problem like tonsillitis. A tonsillectomy will only create a bigger problem in a different part of the child's body. I know a 26 year old man who suffers terrible joint pain since his tonsils were removed. Or a young lady who had her tonsils removed for the repeated tonsillitis and after the surgery, she started ulcerative colitis.

The reason could be emotional and or physical. We will never know unless we look! We certainly do not want anything worse happening to our child by subjecting it to a radical, irreversible surgery. When my daughter was 12 years old her very close friend, Danna, was always sick with tonsillitis. True, she missed many school days, and her mother was burdened by the frequent interruption of job and her daily life routine. Unfortunately, she was administered antibiotics every day for an entire year. Poor Danna, she did not suffer from tonsillitis anymore. Her immune system was so totally shut down through that tetracycline, and with no immune system to fight off disease, Danna died of leukemia at the tender age of 12. Research conducted after her death, not to mention the deaths of many other children who received the same "miraculous" tonsillitis solution, indicated the shocking fact that tetracycline causes leukemia. I do not need to say how shocked and scared all her classmates were. Their trust in the medical establishment and the skills of conventional doctors was shuddered.

All this information surely causes young parents fright and confusion. What does it all have to do with cancer? What can be done if a child has already gone through all of that and then is diagnosed with cancer? Does that mean this child can then only look forward to the prospect of death or lifelong illness? I have even more radical suggestions to address this grave controversy, based on my extensive research through both mainstream and alternative medical authorities and resources.

Every child or adult's body has a mechanism that is constantly on guard. It detects and eradicates every "strange" protein that appears in the body. The goal is quite simply to maintain health. All viruses, bacteria, fungus, etc. are foreign proteins to the body. They simply do not belong to the system; they have no" headquarters" in the brain, unlike every other system in the body. The healthy organism simply has to get rid of those foreign proteins, otherwise they will multiply, take the food and oxygen from the healthy cells and deplete the living body. When the immune system detects a virus cell, bacteria, fungus or even cancer cells, the white blood cells, and lymphatic cells will "consume" it and help the body kick it out. When the "strange cells" are too numerous or too strong, (which can only happen when the body is too weak), the body needs more "fighting" cells in order to complete the job. When these "fighters" multiply and build a "stronger front" the body displays fever, rash, nausea, pain, pus, infection symptoms, and so on. It is not pretty or even comfortable, but it is an important part of the self-healing and life saving process.

Moreover, if we stop or hinder this process, we actually stop the body's self-healing process, and interrupt what the body knows it needs to do. If it happens once or twice, the body gets the message to lay down its arms, as it were, and let the medication fight for it. However, if it frequently recurs and every time the body displays the signs of "battle against an invader" which looks to us and is considered as disease, the body simply "gets the idea" and does not try any more, it can't. It has been disarmed. The body surrenders; it waves the white flag and lets conventional medicine work. The self-healing mechanism has been debilitated and disabled too often by suppressing medications. This happens to people who reach out at the first sneeze or cough to stop the irritation by going to the self-medicating aisle in the supermarket. It is absurd like hiring an outside security guard to watch an army barracks. The body loses its ability to "police" its own health. With the battleground abandoned, this becomes fertile ground for any virus, bacteria and even cancer cells to thrive.

The unhealthy cells thrive under the conditions in which the self-healing mechanism has been paralyzed. With no opposition, they multiply and take over. This is the cancer's path. So, is it true that there is no other way to treat cancer but traditional mainstream medicine? Belief in the traditional way to cut the tumor out, or poison the body with chemotherapy and burn it with radiation is as far from truth as east is from west. It is exactly the other way around. Instead of continuously suppressing the body's immune system, we would be better advised to allow and even encourage the body to regain its immune system and to regain its control over its own life. Sure, that may sound absurd however; the truth is that in many parts of the world these facts have been known for more than 5,000 years now, and even before written history. In ancient Egypt, for instance, cancer-sick people would be treated with hot baths, raising their body's temperature up as high as possible. The reason is; that cancer cells are very sensitive to heat. Cancer cells cannot exist in high temperatures. The high temperature of the body (fever, for example) is deadly for cancer cells. This is exactly what we fight when the child runs a fever. Therefore as you see, fevers are a good sign. In the Dead Sea in Israel, people take very hot sulfur baths. The hot baths elevate the body's temperature to nearly its maximum. This offers tremendous healing properties for all autoimmune disorders. At the Dead Sea, these treatments are recommended for "incurable" skin conditions, as well as all kinds of arthritis which are typical autoimmune deficiency disorders.

The other significant advantage of the Dead Sea is the highly oxygenated air due to the very low elevation (about 360 yards below sea level). A highly oxygenated environment is absolutely deadly for any virus, bacteria, fungus and cancer cell. Where would MEGAForce be if it was widely known that such basic things such as good air was part of the cure for cancer? The proof is in the research labs, where the experiment dishes must be tightly closed, avoiding fresh air (which means, oxygen) from ruining the experiment, when growing a certain virus or bacteria or even cancer cells culture. Does it make any sense to then knock the immune system down with chemotherapy to worsen the body's healthy cells condition, thereby improving the conditions for cancer cells? The main difference between life and disease is –Oxygen. Oxygen is the number one enemy to every cancer cell, or any other foreign protein, like bacteria, fungus, or virus.

Hot geyser springs were used in ancient times for the very same reason: in order to elevate the body temperature supporting and strengthen the immune system so the body can eradicate all unwanted, foreign proteins, including cancer cells.

Think of the traditional sweat lodge of the Native Americans; a tradition stretching back to the very seeds of Native American culture. Or, the sauna in Finland, or the Jacuzzi, the Turkish steam baths, etc., they knew the secret of real health before antibiotics, steroids and chemotherapy were produced by the ruthless pharmaceutical industry. They healed the sick, yet more importantly, they prevented sickness by attending these ceremonies. There is a reason why the Native Americans would honor very special guests by inviting them to their sweat lodge. It is their way to show their respect to their guest, ensuring their guest would leave with optimum health. I should know, since I have experienced it myself.

Traditional healing and cleansing ceremonies have in some way or other included methods of raising the body temperature as high as one can tolerate. I say "as high as one can tolerate" because different constitutions have a different threshold and tolerance for heat, pain, cold, etc. In a meditative state the body can tolerate much higher temperature than it could normally tolerate. Those natural extremes are better for the body than the chemical extremes introduced by the medical establishment.

Can all these ancient traditions be completely wrong and only modern medicine is right? Sorry, but I would rather put my trust in the ancients, who were around for thousands of years. Medical science, meanwhile, is very new. Has modern medicine proved to be successful in healing any disease? I do not mean suppress; I mean heal. Healing means to eradicate the ailment so it never recurs, eradicate WITHOUT any side effects, or a transformation of the problem into a new one that is rooted in the previous disease. This is just medical science playing a shell game. Not one disease has been healed so far by modern medicine. If modern medicine is responsible for anything, it is responsible for diseases being fairly innocuous and acute to being chronic and deadly. I wouldn't really consider that something to be proud of; would you?

As I write this, the FDA has been accused once again for approving a medication for 20 million Americans who suffer from diabetes, which has been found to raise the risk for heart attack by 46 percent and strokes by 61 percent. The reason is nothing new, and should come as no surprise to even the most naive: The FDA is a cabal of drug makers and pharmaceutical manufacturers who have the power to create the law because they have congress pretty much in their pocket. Approving a medication means that the manufacturers will make millions, sure, but it goes beyond that. Others will make even more, because the side effects will force the poor people who are seeking a "cure"- to need more medications to deal with the side effects, and meanwhile the industry around it is thriving. So, what would be their incentive NOT to approve such deadly medications?

However, despite many years of research showing its efficiency, pulsed electromagnetic field therapy, a healing method used all over the world, is banned in America because the FDA flat out refuses to approve it. The FDA knows very

Giggling Dr. Green

well why it had better not approve it, because it is bad for the bottom line of MEGA Force. There is not much money to be made in this healing method. People only have to purchase one device that lasts them as long as 20-25 years, which can be used by the whole family. Such a device would save millions from being victimized by the FDA and the mainstream medical establishment.

Moreover, we all fall into that same trap. We all must stop this vicious circle of insane greed and the dance of death, a dance we perform only for the sake of their greed. We all must help our kids. They are our highest value. We must get them back to their natural state of health, their state of freedom.

Do you know that a person who has been diagnosed with cancer could recover within a few weeks simply through vegetable juices, green leafy rich diet, fermented vegetables relaxation, exercise, guided visionary therapy, water and fresh air? Maybe some reflexology treatments, and possibly pulse electromagnetic therapy? That is all we need. Had I not seen it time and again in these past 43 years, I would not believe it myself, perhaps as you still do not. Nevertheless, whether you accept it or not, it is food for thought that can save millions of lives of both adults and children, and maybe, your own child as well.

It was the summer of 1987, when a young woman came into my office. She wore a scarf on her head. Although she was very pretty, you could see in her eyes and her skin how sick she was; there was deadness and grayness to her. She told me that she had been diagnosed with leukemia and that she had been treated with chemotherapy, that her prognosis was very chilling. She was scared, like everyone would be, and even more so because she was very young with two babies at home. She asked for my help as she trembled while speaking; "They missed my vein and the chemo ran into my arm muscle, so the burning pain is unbearable. They couldn't help me," she added. I did not leap up and offer her a miracle cure. In fact, I was very apprehensive and wondered whether there would be anything I could do with homeopathy that could at least alleviate her burning pain. Nonetheless, I mustered my best resources and gave her a homeopathic remedy. On her way out she gave me a pleading look and said, "Please don't tell my husband I was here. You know, he is very much against people like you." I said okay, and never heard from her again. Judging by her ashen complexion and prognosis, things quite frankly looked absolutely hopeless.

Seventeen years later I heard from that lady. She told me she was in perfect health and did not receive any more chemotherapy after the homeopathic remedy, because there were no leukemia indications in her blood to be found anymore.

Giggling Dr. Green

I am not telling this story to brag about how a certain remedy or treatment can work a miracle. Rather, it is to show you how many healing possibilities are out there: There are so many wonderful, simple, natural, non-invasive, harmless methods that can be absolutely life saving. After all, cancer is like many other chronic dies-eases, and takes a long time to heal.

Suggestions for prevention and healing

Here are a few suggestions for keeping up your health, whether you are battling disease or wisely want to avoid getting sick.

Vegetable juice fasting. This can be carried out for a whole month if necessary.

After the tumor has shrunk or completely disappears, please do not resume your old diet. This can prove disastrous, and may put you back where you started! Please let your child learn to eat healthy food only. Remember, children learn what they live, far better than they will ever learn what you set out to teach them. Live your life before them in the way you desire to see them living, and the entire family will benefit in marvelous ways.

The preferred vegetables would be carrots, celery, beets, kale, spinach, sweet potatoes, Green apple, and lemon with the white pith. Drinking five cups of this wonderful raw elixir daily could make a huge breakthrough.

My other suggestion would be to stay away, completely, from any animal protein. Yes, that means no meat, chicken, eggs, ham, cheese, milk, fish, during this important season. No sugar or any baked goods, no bread. No processed food. Just raw vegetables, brown rice and water. Apple cider vinegar, at least twice a day,(on one glass of water, 1 tablespoon Apple cider vinegar, and 6-10 drops of Stevia could be added), will be helpful. Spend time outdoors in the fresh air and direct sun. Moreover, let's not forget the other ingredients: lots of laughter and joy should be the most important part of the day. A lot of love, warmth and support. Drawing and painting all the thoughts, fears and concerns away. Plenty of physical activity, but without any undue strain and exertion. Plenty of sleep. Make sure that things like school demands and success are not even mentioned, let alone considered as important as the healing time. Conversation with the child is necessary. Let him or her know that it is safe to say and express anything, even if it may hurt someone (not on purpose, of course). Please be aware that all this expressiveness is not just good for the soul, it is absolutely vital for the body to heal itself.

Giggling Dr. Green

Music is also an important part in healing. The child should either be encouraged to sing or listen to very soothing, comforting and pleasant music, to dance and play. Just simply change everything that was dysfunctional in the child's life into functionality. If parents are divorced and it really had an impact on the child, please reassure your child that it had nothing to do with him or her, and be sure to express how much you love him or her. Let the child tell you everything that scares or bathers him or her.

Just as many wild animals feel threatened and frightened in captivity and therefore get very sick, so do our children. Children must have the proper conditions to simply be happy. It is not complicated; it does not take much. No fancy house is needed, nor are luxury cars; no expensive clothes or toys are necessary to make a child happy. It does, however, require a healthy emotional relationship based on love, and regular encouragement and opportunity to establish good relationships with other children, as well as nature and animals. We do not need more than just very simple food and a simple bed. What else do we really need in order to be happy? Yes, one more important thing is - freedom. I mean also freedom of drugs, anything suppressive that takes our basic freedom of functioning and thriving, away.

Healing nutrition makes sense

This diet creates a "protein starvation". If the body gets no animal protein for an extended period of time, but only plant protein something miraculous happens. First off, plant protein is a simpler protein chain. It leaves no toxic residues like the animal protein does. The kidneys have significantly fewer struggles breaking these residues down and eliminating them from the body. The plants are cancer's worst enemy because they enrich the cells with what are now known as phyto-chemicals that are virtually deadly to the cancer cells. A phyto-chemical is a natural bioactive compound found in plant foods that works with nutrients and dietary fiber to protect against disease. Tremendous research shows that phyto-chemicals, working together with the naturally healthy nutrients found in fruits, vegetables and nuts, help to slow the aging process and reduce the risk of many diseases, including cancer, heart disease, stroke, high blood pressure, cataracts, osteoporosis, and urinary tract infections and so many more. The word is pronounced 'fight-o- chemicals'! What a wonderful way to remember that eating this way, as a lifestyle, is like sending in legions of marines to aid your body in fighting off disease.

The healthy cells light up due to the chlorophyll from the green vegetables, which cancer cells and all other disease proteins don't have.

Giggling Dr. Green

The "antioxidant" environment is also deadly to cancer cells. What the cancer cells truly need is very highly acidic blood, a very poorly oxygenated body; it needs animal protein and a lot of sugar, a very low electromagnetic field, and very low positive microflora in the intestines. All these are absolutely necessary for the cancer cells to thrive. The animal protein starvation process creates the exact opposite conditions. Once starved of animal protein, the body will then start to search and consume any "strange" protein inside itself. Without animal protein the need will become so crucial that the body will start to "look for" protein in every possible "old storage area" in the body and will start to consume the cancer cells, since these are "considered" by the body as foreign proteins.

The energy level will rise significantly. The digestion system is demanding up to 80% of the body's energy. See how people are warned not to drive after a saturating meal for their security on the road. Driver's awareness diminishes after a rich meal. We can also see how many people need a little nap after their meal. The energy the body needs for digestion is high, especially when meat or any animal protein is served. When the food is made of just fresh vegetables, the body needs less energy for digestion. This "extra" energy the body will use for the healing process. Healing also takes a lot of energy, and therefore it is why I emphasize plenty of rest and sleep. The sleep helps the body to recover the hemoglobin level in the blood as well as enrich the blood with oxygen. Since the muscles rest throughout the sleep, the energy will then be directed to the vital organs for the healing process

If it worked for thousands of people, it can probably work for you as well. Does that seem overly simplified? I bet it does. Yet, nature in its infinite beauty is very simple. Like

Dr. Gannot said to me many years ago, "Every time I listen to you, I translate all you said in simple words, into science vocabulary, on my way home. I am amazed how true everything I heard from you was, and how we, for so many years, find all this information in our research, yet, never find a way to simply apply it in the manner you suggest." Since treating him for his very severe health problems, I have seen and treated so many more people in my very "simplified" ways. With significant success rates, thank God.

There has been a very dangerous trend in the past 60 years concerning proteins. After World War II, protein became not only very popular but an obsession. Nutrition experts thought that protein was the most important part in our nutrition. It is true, but only partially. If we know how every cell is built, we know how important the protein is for the cells. However, we fail to appreciate the fact that the body creates its most important protein, as well as the power and potency of plant protein as well. A diet does not need to be centered on animal protein.

Like one of my clients said to me, "I can't forget that you said how you don't eat anything that had eyes or a mother." We also forget that meat products as well as dairy products are made of very sick, undernourished animals, animals that are raised under the most cruel and gruesome conditions. How healthy can that food be? Research has shown that the fear and anxiety related hormones an animal secretes into its blood, is real poison to the consumer of their meat. In addition, remember that everything the animals eat, we eat too. Are you aware of the "food" the animals get? Thus, we do get the same hormones and medications that the livestock gets through the meat and animal-derived food we eat. These poor animals, had they not been slaughtered in time, would not be allowed on the market because of the cancers and all the other diseases they would be soon displaying. This alone is probably a very significant factor for so much disease.

Please read the book <u>Diet for a New America</u> by John Robbins. It will make you reconsider ever touching meat again, not to mention giving it to your children.

Farmed fish are also a big nutritional problem, because these poor fish are fed and medicated as bad as the animal for meat and dairy production.

We all know how it says that "mothers should not have alcohol and cigarettes when they are pregnant and nurse". Well, the dairy and milk producers do not really care that all the hormones and medications the livestock receives go straight into our children's blood.

All these should be out of every child's diet, but absolutely banned from every sick child diet and for chronic disease health processes as well.

When Todd called me a few years ago he said, "I know that I don't have much time left, yet one thing I have learned is that, had I not had health insurance, I would have stayed alive longer, and been healthier longer." This may sound ludicrous, but please allow me to explain. He had cancer and went through all the medical procedures because he was insured and received many "treatments free". How ironic! Only later on he learned how simple juice fasting, reflexology, homeopathy, pulsed electromagnetic field therapy, guided imagery or visualization, and exercise would probably turn the wheel around for him.

Cancer cells are really not the evil they are made out to be. The body produces them when for some reason the right programming goes astray. The right thing to do would be to help the "right programming", go right again, which means correction of the immune system functioning and in so doing, prevent the mistaken and aberrant cell production. It is not much different in children's bodies. The many medications, vaccinations, or very unhealthy food, and/or emotional stress, can cause a grave error in the cell's production system. If we just correct the cause, the body will do everything it possibly can to correct itself and its own functions. There is nothing, absolutely nothing, stronger than the living organism's drive for life. This is the strongest drive of every living creature, every human being, every animal and every plant. There is nothing that any living creature would invest more effort and more energy in than in maintaining life. Therefore, I suggest that you take a proactive role in helping your child's body to keep and maintain life. Helping means not interfering and not disrupting its basic processes. Just support it, and you will be amazed how wonderful nature is at fighting for its life.

Does it make any sense, that deadly poison could maintain life?

Have you ever wondered what chemotherapy entails: what the ingredients are? Can life continue by killing parts of it off? Is it possible that by trying to "kill" cells that the body has built itself, that health can be restored? Can a body, that for some reason has given up and "chose" death, be revived by poisons? If a child sees his parents separate and is very scared and desperate, and even feels guilty, can he be consoled and comforted by surgery and chemicals? It is simply not possible; to believe so is lunacy. I believe that if our joy of life has been taken away from us and the body starts to shut down, that means that our "life force" has been shut down. Only a huge smile, healthy food, emotional support, and learning how to cope with the emotional pain would be the way to health.

I have seen so much fear, pain and unnecessary death. On the other hand, I also have seen so much new light, promise and success in healing. Like little Edoh who had a very aggressive cancer, Neuroblastoma,

He has been fighting this disease since he was just 3 years old. He went through many chemotherapy sessions as well as radiation. Edoh spent many days and months in the hospital, and the doctors told his parents there was nothing left to do for him anymore. With just some simple pulse electromagnetic therapy sessions, he started to heal and recover. He was sent home from the hospital with no further answers; it had to be terrifying for a tiny child and even more for his family. He had a few more weeks to live and he was just 6 years old. His parents took a leap of faith since they had no other choice or options left. In addition, thanks to alternative therapies, Edoh continued to get better year after year in spite of the prognosis. Had his parents just listened to the physicians, Edoh would have died at the age of six. Isn't this the saddest thing any parent could face? However, if you still think that I am simplifying the dreadful cancer to ridiculous degree, do not take my advice on blind faith; walk the path you believe is the right path for your child. All I bring you in this book are different possible ways not prescriptions for what to do, but just sharing my thoughts, knowledge and experience. Sometimes, it is true; I have been confronted by angry skeptics who would happily hang me for my thinking. On the other hand, many people's lives have been saved by this advice as well. Therefore, it is your choice.

Electromagnetic field therapy

EMF is a very low frequency which is the earth magnetic field. It has been proved to stimulate healthy cell metabolism.

Whenever I try to explain how EMF works, I realize that not everyone is an expert in biology, or electromagnetic low-frequency field therapy. There are not even many mainstream doctors who grasp the idea. It does not belong to the known world of Newtonian physics; rather, it is quantum physics. Notice; this experimenting and research of quantum physics, had begun long before Einstein's discoveries, who by the way, was a very devoted fan of these theories. In the past century, these theories emerged to the dismay of many scientists who could accept only Newton's physics known so far and have been used for many different purposes among them, therapy. In mainstream medicine, these low-frequency waves are used for example in MRI machines. In America, which is known for its vigorous FDA resistance to alternative and complementary medicine of any kind, people have demanded the right to use the EMF therapy. Even the FDA has allowed EMF therapy into mainstream medical facilities for bone fusion and bone loss therapy. For many years people only "believed" that Mozart music has some kind of beneficial influence on children's brain development. For the past 25 years (even longer in France), science has proved the reasoning behind that assumption, and many institutes already use Mozart's fine music to enhance and strengthen children's development with proven results, as the resonance of that music is the leading note for this notion.

The same goes for EMF therapy. Though it is not the same as Mozart's wonderful music, the commonality is the positive impact it has on a living organism's health and wellness, through nothing but mild waves.

These waves stimulate the cell metabolism. When cell metabolism becomes activated, the cells start to eliminate waste and absorb and assimilate the nutrients and oxygen. Under this influence the molecules actively start to produce the ATP which is the protein that is the vital energy source for the cell proper functioning for all vital processes.

To describe it in a more visual way, let me tell you a little story about the cells. Cells are the building blocks of our material being, that is, our physical body. However, wherever there are good cells, e.g. our healthy cells, there are also "bad" cells hanging around, that may blossom into disease if not eliminated. It is simply the job of the healthy cells to consume the bad cells (dead cells and foreign proteins for example), and keep the body clean of these potent harmful cells. Now, these unhealthy cells do not necessarily come from outside. Believe it or not, we produce most of them ourselves. When the healthy cell's life span is up, it dies off and new healthy cells emerge. Meanwhile, the bad cells are wasted in the body; they turn into lifeless protein that needs to be expelled. Thus, the "healthy cells" are not always exactly healthy and if they are not really healthy, they are unable to "consume" and transfer the dead cells or the bad cells out of the system; or, in another scenario, they cannot metabolize efficiently, or cannot bind oxygen sufficiently. They may simply act like us when we are not healthy. You know how it is when you cannot go to work or play as easily as you do when you are healthy. Therefore, we need to make sure that the healthy cells are actually healthy. The unhealthy cells are those we would call viruses, bacteria, fungus, cancer, etc. or, simply "dysfunctional cells." If they are dysfunctional, they will lower the efficiency of the body's natural ability to maintain and preserve its basic functions. This is disease in its simplest definition.

Look at it this way; healthy cells are like our mirror. A body with plenty of healthy cells will be displaying vibrant health, excellent blood work results, good energy level, not too high, or too low. In addition, the bowel movements are natural and consistent; the urination will be good in color, consistency and frequency. The skin will look fresh and radiant, as well as the hair. The eyes look clear, lively, and full of sparkle and light. The state of mind will be positive, outgoing, enthusiastic, confident, tolerant and happy. The brain will be functioning at top capacity, lively and alert. There will be no offensive body odor of any kind. There will not be any anxiety or undue stress. The appetite will be very good and natural, not overly hungry, and also with no aversion to eating, just naturally strong.

In summary, this is the optimal picture of health, and our cells should be as healthy on the inside as we look on the outside (not smiling and happy, necessarily, but you know what I mean!). Furthermore, the cells need to be doing all this "work" without any special effort. Thus, when all the healthy cells are healthy, their job of contributing to our overall health should not be terrifically difficult. That means that the immune system is functioning good and efficiently. That means that the "poor" unhealthy cells cannot thrive and are quickly disposed of. You see, the difference between the healthy and unhealthy cells is in the "living conditions" each of them needs. It is like us humans; healthy, happy people who love their life, who nurture their health and enjoy their work, will thrive in a healthy, well-ventilated, non-polluted environment, with healthy food choices, while maintaining a balanced weight. Unhealthy people cannot stand this environment. People who do not care about their health, are unhappy in their job, and do not respect their lives in general, will feel very uncomfortable in a healthy environment, be intolerant, grumpy, grouchy, with offensive body odors. It is almost toxic to them and they are for their surroundings. The same goes for healthy and unhealthy cells. The healthy cells thrive on healthy food, an oxygen-rich environment, a well-functioning metabolism, and a proper electromagnetic field. Unhealthy cells need a much lower electromagnetic field frequency; furthermore, they cannot stand oxygen at all, and healthy food is deadly for them because it has too many antioxidants, too much oxygen and too many phytochemicals. All those components are simply deadly for them. The pulse electromagnetic field therapy has such a powerfully positive effect on the human body. The main differences between health and disease are oxygen and metabolism. In an oxygen-rich environment, no unhealthy cells can survive. The only differences between life and death are- oxygen and metabolism. In other words, if we can create a condition in which the healthy cells are able to bind with as much oxygen as they possibly can absorb, we help the body; we help it heal and release the waste by creating health-enhancing conditions. This is what EMF therapy does. When it comes down to it, it really does not matter what the name or label of any given disease is. Health is simply a hearty metabolism and sufficient oxygen absorption. Disease occurs when the conditions allow the opposite. Just as health is a combination of more than just one condition, so disease is a combination of many different factors that disable and disrupt health. The body itself with the proper support can easily heal cancer simply by stopping it.

Why do drugs never work?

This has been probably the biggest question in our lifetime. Since pharmacists discovered the art of medicine, the never-ending search for new drugs continues to bring new drugs to the market every day. The basic concept of drugs for health disappeared years ago, yet today the drug market is the strongest and most prosperous market in the world. Even more than food.

Giggling Dr. Green

Using drug preparations began when man first discovered the healing properties of different plants.

People in the most remote and primitive tribes knew how to use different plants for various ailments and disorders. At that time, in their arts of healing, they did not label diseases other than naming the very obvious symptoms. For example "angry liver" or "guilty kidney." In time, the pharmaceutical industry developed into a huge market and money making concern like every other commercialized market.

The essence of drugs continued to be plant-derived products. Take, for instance, aspirin, morphine, and valium and so on. The difference between the synthetic medications made by the pharmaceutical companies and the natural herb or animal derived product is how the medications are chosen and processed. The natural medications were chosen by how their effects resemble the symptoms. For example: when the patient would run a very high fever, would look very angry, blushed, and would have an aversion to water, the possible plant resembling the Belladonna fruit . This fruit is extremely toxic in its natural form, however, if the healer would take just a tiny little portion of the fruit, and would let the patient, let's say, just smell it, the body would receive the resembling message, the very message of the healing properties, and would respond by calming down. Natural medications, which are called "remedies", in order to keep set apart from the medications made by pharmaceutical companies, release a very subtle aroma, through their essential oils. That aroma sends a stimulating message that resembles the very same reaction to the body's cells as the body is already displaying. Since two similar diseases cannot exist in the body at the same time (via Dr Samuel Hahnemann), the body will experience the "same" disease in a very weak form. That will stimulate the self-healing agents in the body and will help the body heal itself. If the body overcomes that "smelled irritant" it becomes able to overcome the original disease.

This is the way naturopathic medicine works to help the patient overcome his ailments. By pushing the symptoms away, via the traditional allopathic medicine approach, we will never be able to recover long lasting, truly stable health. The proof is in the pudding. See the "recurring" diseases so many people suffer from? In many cases children whose parents have to struggle with recurring tonsillitis, strep, sinus issues, bladder infections, or skin rashes etc… The reason for the chronic incidents is only that; the body never had a chance to overcome them by itself. Medicine always did the job for them, or seemed to.

Giggling Dr. Green

This idea is somewhat related to the general idea of vaccinations. When the body receives a vaccination, it should be able to "learn" through the inoculated weakened agent to deal with and heal the specific disease. The difference between these two approaches is that when a disease happens naturally and the body receives all the support it needs to "fight" it, the body will be able to develop the antibodies. How? By running a high fever, by creating pus or swellings, vomiting, loss of appetite, rash, itchy, red eyes, cough etc. all the signs of what we call disease. However, when the vaccinations are given, the disease agent, whether it is a virus, bacteria or fungus, is so weak that the body cannot develop the normal resisting mechanisms such as high fever, vomiting or diarrhea. The stimulation is insufficient or none. However, in order to have sufficient stimulation, the risk is too high in unleashing the disease in its full magnitude, and it could put the patient in danger. The terrible "accidents" that so many children suffer from after receiving vaccinations are visible proof. Because the body could not really fight all the diseases in the vaccination, the immune system remains harmed, disabled and many times seriously impaired for the rest of their lives.

The other reason for complications arising from vaccines is that many different agents, poisons, really, are inoculated into the body at the same time. This would cause an absolute deadly reaction had the disease agents been even just the smallest fraction stronger than they are. The natural remedies, however, are based on a plant's natural essential oils, specific fluid combinations; certain assets the plants have that stimulate the expected reaction in the body. Take for instance the aloe vera plant. This plant is one of the most health-promoting plants, due to the very special and yes, somewhat slimy fluids in its branches. The aloe vera leaves we know are in fact their branches, and the thorns are the leaves. Just think how huge natural pharmacies in our world are available for use instead of the poisons of the so-called medications.

When it comes to classic homeopathy, people ask, "Do you have something to use against headaches"? My answer will always be no. Because there is nothing in classic homeopathy that is actually "against" anything. Classic homeopathy is based upon observation and finding the remedy that would create similar, typical, unusual reactions in the body, if the remedy were to be admitted in larger amounts. The difference between natural medicine and allopathic medicine is in the approach. Do we want to stop the symptoms through numbing the body? Alternatively, do we want to help the body address the original cause that created that specific problem? When we choose to numb the symptoms, eventually we are creating a chronic disease. Since the deeper reason has never been addressed and the body never got the opportunity to actively fight the problem, or actively restore balance, the problem will always remain in the body. By attempting to cut out the problem with surgery, or further poison it through chemotherapy or other means, we actually cause the body to find different "alleys" through which to fight for its life - before resigning. We then face the known complications, or new disease name - metastasized cells.

Does it sound strange when we say that by creating cancer the body is actually fighting for life? We have been programmed to think about cancer as the mainstream medical wants us to think, which is: Cancer has to be removed because it threatens life. The truth is the exact opposite. The truth is; the body "concentrates" the unhealthy cells it cannot expel, into one tumor. This tumor is actually indicating that the immune system is at its wit's end. The wise way to treat the problem here would be to enhance the immune system and restore the self-healing assets through it. Yet, the allopathic medicine establishment thinks very differently, and we all know how that goes: It begins the battle with chemotherapy. If the tumor has been removed, and the lymphatic nodes have been removed as well, what will be left for the body to heal itself with now? How does removing the lymph nodes help to restore health? People who were diagnosed with cancer who desire to keep all their lymph nodes are much better able to restore their own health because they still have the necessary glands to transport the lymphatic fluid, a basic tool of the body to heal itself.

If cancer has been diagnosed in a person and the doctor would spend the time to inquire into the previous year or two in that patient's life, he would be able to discover what triggered this total collapse of the life force in that person. The other step should be restoration of the life force by strengthening the immune system and modifying his lifestyle. However, the "traditional way" is to see cancer as "the bad guy" and then we deploy the cannons to "kill it." Don't we realize that this way we kill the person along with the cancer? The only true way to restore health is to support the body to actively use its natural self-healing mechanism.

Only in very severe cases in which the life force is so depleted would chemical drugs ever be considered helpful. However, it is not as a means to heal disease, most certainly not in recurrent cases. As a rule, no medication should be used for an acute, or long-term illness, and for any other reason but to help to save lives that are in immediate grave danger. Certainly should never be used primarily to promote the drug industry and fatten its bottom line.

So, why would the pharmaceutical industry turn these healing plants into chemical products? Why wouldn't they simply leave them in their natural state and serve the herbs instead of the manufactured chemical products? They could probably come up with many different answers, but at least a few of the more truthful ones are as obvious as the nose on your face. For instance, preserving the drugs to last longer on the market. Another reason is; this way they are more convenient to use and market them. It is unnecessary to search for the plant, find the right one and prepare it to be used to heal. I guess the basic idea behind the pharmaceutical drugs preparations was very good, helpful and necessary in the early days. Think about the famous Chinese herbs that are prepared in pill form so all one needs to do is just open the container and pour five pills into the hand, and with a glass of water pop them in. But the Chinese herbs still keep their natural odor, and you can actually detect the combination of the pills by smelling them.

Western medicine pills have hardly any odor and are colorful, tasty and sugar coated, in order to appeal to kids. This teaches children to love and become dependent on medications which turns them into addicts when they grow up. Unfortunately the pharmaceutical industry is as commercial as any other financial oriented industry. Pharmacology has moved away from the original medicine of men and women in the primitive tribes, who prepared their potions and elixirs to heal the sick people. The pharmaceutical companies thrived in their business and made men dependent upon their products in an outrageous success. Within the past century, these companies became a world leading financial power, from the typical person seeking a cold remedy to the halls of congress. Now, those of us who try to fight off brainwashing as; every disease has to have a name, every disease has a drug, every disease must be stopped, diseases are epidemics and life threatening. The irony is that we are called alternative medicine practitioners or complementary medicine practitioners. Isn't this the opposite of the truth? Doesn't it seem terribly odd to you? How is it conceivable that the original has now become the alternative and the artificial has now been deemed mainstream? Because we allow it to be. Because we allowed the pharmaceutical companies to take over and dictate our health, to force us to use debilitating and poisonous drugs. They do not do it for our health and well-being.

We keep our ignorance rather than educate ourselves for our own protection. It is a sort of immune system deficiency - we keep the fertile ground for those scavengers as we don't feel knowledgeable and sufficiently educated to fight them and to prove them wrong and reclaim our right and ability to good health and life.

So, why do drugs never work? Drugs are made of chemicals, or, in the best-case scenario, derived from animal hormones or organs, or synthetic hormones and imitations of plants healing properties. I do not get into all the details of what drugs are made of, because I basically resent the whole drug concept and industry. Nevertheless, this is my personal opinion. When we get a very bad headache, for example could it be an indication of Tylenol deficiency? Could cancer be an indication of chemotherapy, radiation or surgery deficiency? The sick person has become off balance, this is what we see as disease. As it is called -dis-ease. Only if the reason for the imbalance be it due to trauma, prolonged stress conditions, food intolerance, grief or any other reason is known - healing can take place.

In fact, intense headache, migraines and constipation can be correlated. Spine misalignment can be the source for indigestion. Headaches could be the result of bad shoes, as the tonsillitis can be caused by neck muscles hypertension.

With allopathic medicine, the medications create a chemical reaction to suppress the symptoms. Has any healing taken place? Isn't it like when the red light on the car dashboard comes on, signaling an engine problem, and we just disable the red light bulb. Would that solve our engine problems? Of course not, the engine would burn up!

I was listening to a radio talk show one Saturday morning, when mechanics answered car issues questions. A lady asked the mechanics if it might be possible that driving several hundred miles with tape over the oil pressure light, could have been related to the engine braking down. Is this funny? Well, we do the same with Tylenol and all other signal suppressing medications.

The kidney must be able to identify the medicine in order to process these chemicals, so they will accumulate in the kidney, or may "travel" with the bloodstream to accumulate in different body parts, since no one was born with a chemical lab index to know how to deal with the chemicals. Just as the food coloring, the preservatives and all the other artificial additives in processed food. The kidney is just one of the different organs to deal with the chemical agents administered to the body, in order to "solve" the problem they created. Don't we then create a new problem? Well, if we create a new problem, is it after we dealt with the first problem or is it added on top of the original problem? Well, you are right if you suspected it only adds to the original problem, making things worse than they already were. So, if this is the case, why do we allow anyone to talk us into the vicious circles that always end up either in crippling or killing us?

So, why don't drugs work? There are countless reasons, two of which I will mention here:

1. If they would actually work, the patients would get well, and that would cause a major recession.

Giggling Dr. Green

2. Because suppression creates just more need for drugs and medical procedures - healthy for the economy.

I like to alert parents to start and change these monstrous rules of a greed-driven industry that has no values and is nothing short of drug dealers and pushers to whom your child's life means nothing as long as business is prosperous. Get the information and make healthy choices.

The power of visualization

Alice was lying in her bed, both hands holding her stomach and tears running down her cheeks. She cried for quite a while and the pain was not letting up at all. The doctor was supposed to pay her a visit. Her mother came into her room, with a look in her eyes as if she had seen the worst disaster ever, by looking into her little girl's eyes.

Her mother's concerned look reflected to Alice that something must be terribly wrong with her stomach, or else, why would her mother look so worried? Alice crying got even worse. The poor, anxiety-ridden mother could not muster even one comforting word for her beloved daughter and Alice realized that she must be seriously ill, if the mother was in a state of such despair.

After the doctor's examination, the mother felt a significant relief and managed to squeeze a smile through her tears. The prognosis was that in two or three days Alice would be completely well. It was nothing serious and a simple homemade application would help the young child.

Years later, when Alice was in her twenties and became ill again she demanded her mother to stay out of her room before she was well. She said; "I could never forget the fear in my mother's eyes whenever I got sick as a child. Mother's anguish had always created so much additional tension and fear, I could actually feel myself getting worse and worse by the minute. However, when mother would finally smile, I would feel better right away."

Had Alice's mother been more aware, she would have understood that every sick child draws his courage, hope, support and power to overcome, from his parents. I cannot forget my own mother's look when I was sick. I dreaded her presence when I was ill, because I felt even as a child how instead of drawing strength from her, my strength was depleted by her. Just by worrying she transmitted it to me without even one word. The feelings I sensed from my own mother were of that danger, disaster, death, fear, suffering, helplessness and hopelessness. When a child is sick, all it needs are some beautiful, well-loved old stories that would carry it away on a beautiful imaginary trip to a world of beauty, light, hope, health, play, laughter, and painlessness. It does not cost us anything to take that trip with our child. Remember the picture of the little child laughing through his tears? This is an unbelievably powerful tool to help the child to find the inner strength and hope whenever times of adversity in his little life. It should be added in the "Home pharmacy" chapter and not just for our children but for us as adults as well. I have been in a huge conflict with the mainstream approach when it says: "The patient must hear the truth." My question is what is the truth? Who can say that what the doctors think they know is really the truth?

When I broke my foot as I ran up the stairs, when I visited my sister, her response was: "See, this is typical for a country girl who doesn't know how to use the elevator." Instead of feeling sorry for myself, and in spite of my pain, I had to laugh at the way she treated me, and the pain seemed to lessen. She did not display her anxiety and worry about me. This is almost a tradition in our family. We all keep our sense of humor when visiting or treating each other, no matter how serious the condition may look. So far, it has always worked wonders.

The secret of visualization works best with children, but is very beneficial with adults as well. The problem is that we listen to the horrible news the doctors and tests tell us, and forget that no one knows the deepest secrets of nature. Nature has so many more amazing surprises in store for us to overcome, than we could ever imagine. The incredible power of nature is really only understood on a very superficial level by even the finest minds science has to offer. There are boundless secrets hidden in nature, and often, for those who choose to live in harmony with all that grows and breathes life, will have a deeper understanding of what is good and worthy, more than all the books could ever teach us. We may never know nearly as much as we would like to know. One thing that everyone can agree with - when it comes to the magnificent world of nature, so much more we do not know than what we do know. When worried over a sick child, by empowering and helping the child to "ride on the imaginary horse" to its mystical wonderland, we provide him with the most precious medicine ever.

Inner Secretes are our healing hormones

The way our inner self healing mechanism truly works is by secretion of the necessary hormones into the bloodstream. For instance, the adrenalin in case of injury or threat, or extra exertion, runs for life, competition. The insulin to utilize the sugar, or, endorphin to relax and calm down pain. Many other hormones run through our blood and every hormone has its importance. The "guide" to direct the hormones is thought to be the brain. (Not all scientists agree completely on this). When the brain detects imminent danger it will signal the adrenal gland to release more adrenaline into the blood for the heart to pump faster, so the legs can run faster, and even the intestines evacuate its contents to "make it easier" for the body to flee. Like trained athletes who are very sensitive to the "go" gun at track, so are we very sensitive to good or bad news. When you are at the doctor's office and hear him say: "good afternoon Mr. Smith, please be seated. I am sorry, but I have very bad news for you"…..this same moment your body has an internal reaction within seconds. The blood starts to rush and you can feel your heart race, the stomach "turns" and you feel you want to throw up, you feel a cold sweat covers your whole body, you feel how your blood leaves your face and feel faint and have not heard what the doctor had to tell you yet. The same can happen in the complete opposite way. Imagine that your phone rings. You pick it up and your little girl screams out loud that she is finally back from her long absence during which you were extremely worried about her. The same instance, your heart starts to pump very fast; you feel how the tears of happiness and thankfulness to the divine fill your eyes. You start dancing with the phone still in your hand and right away get ready to pick her up.

In both occasions the brain sent the message to the hormone glands to secrete the needed hormones into the blood. This is how positive energy, visualization, imagination, gentle touch, laughter and joy send the message to the brain to pour the vitally important hormones into the blood. Yet, unlike the time of bad news the body secretes the vitalizing hormones that actually promptly replenish the immune system and self-healing ability. The life force takes over immediately.

This is how it always has and always will work.

We reveal to the child the key to his own inner power, to the life force that can overcome everything, just because it is stronger than any medicine, or any pain, stronger than any virus, or bacterium. After all, this is the only true power that created us in the first place. This is the true power that plays the role when "miraculously" a person recovers from the brink of a deadly condition. In the Schneider Children's Hospital, in Israel, the proof is in the pudding, when clowns are part of the staff and medical procedures. It has been scientifically proven that the healing process is faster and better when the children are able to laugh and have fun. I am living proof of that as well. In the most horrible moments, I could take an internal position of strength and decide to fight and never give in. In the worst bout of suffering, I could hear my inner self smile and say, "Hey, we can do it! Just hang in there! They don't know what nature knows!" And you know what? It worked, it really did. It took me three years to get well, (in spite of the doctor's prognosis that I had just three more weeks to live) but it was worth it just to use the inner power of my own mind. The mind is able to make these decisions. Children can learn this little secret and thrive on it always, under any circumstances. The same results children achieve through painting and craft, since it is so vital for their creative imagination to heal and stay well.

When Ab was diagnosed with leukemia, the doctors said it was a hopeless case, and he was sent home to die. Well, Ab chose not to accept the grim prognosis, and his wise family agreed with him. He decided he had the will and power to ignore the death sentence, reach into his deeply seated life force, and turn the wheel around. Like so many others, he succeeded. Instead of accepting the limits of modern medicine, he told me how he turned around to ignore and disregard everything he heard and just put all his trust in the universal power and his inner life force that told him; "Simply synchronize," as he explained later. If we can learn this secret that has never been taught in medical schools, we can give our children and ourselves the greatest gift ever, one that will sustain them and us throughout. I had been there myself several times and taught my children as well as my grandchildren this beautiful tool that we can all use; the "medical miracle maker" that cannot be bought in any pharmacy nor is it taught in any medical school. It is not even subject to FDA approval or regulation and it cannot be found in any medicine bottle; it is solely our own wonderful treasure. No one can buy it for us; no one can give it or take it away from us. It is our inborn power and all we need is to learn how to access it when we are in need of its ability to speak calmly into the storm.

Whenever a child gets sick or hurts, it is time for us to reach out for the power that lies within us, sending positive energy to the child. If we cry, especially in the child's presence, or obsess about potential danger that lies ahead or even think of it, we are disempowering the child, and actually bring further negativity into an already difficult situation. Young children are not highly educated; however they understand and believe that we must know more than they do. Our demeanor will greatly influence our child's ability to draw on nature as a tool for inner healing. Children are so wonderfully sensitive and capable of actually feeling the vibrations of energy around them, whether positive or negative. In this sense they are very much like an animal that senses danger without exactly realizing it. When a deadly storm, such as a tsunami, is still quite a distance off and before anyone has any knowledge of the impending disaster, all the animals will disappear from that area before the calamity strikes. Children are so very similar due to their young, unspoiled intuitive instincts. They have not yet

Giggling Dr. Green

discovered what impossible means. If they are fortunate with parents who teach them to always reach for the stars, they never will learn to limit themselves.

By nature, children have marvelous abilities to detect any vibrations, messages and thoughts without any conscious effort. They simply understand at a deeper level than we may give them credit for. When sitting at the child's bed, the best thing we can do is train our mind to think positive. If you have any concern or doubt, please take a moment before entering the sick child's room and clear your thoughts. Train your mind to keep hope and a good sense of humor at the forefront of all you do. The child's little invisible "antenna" will pick up on it immediately causing her or his heart to swell with courage, power, hope, and positive feelings which will empower his life force. In case of sickness, the chances for recovery are doubled and tripled in a way you may find difficult to believe, before it becomes your way of life. After all, as the quantum physicists know already, energy is an ongoing flow; energy never stops and never lessens. Energy is invisible yet transforms everything and anything.

Thoughts are the seed of manifestation; even the bible confirms it. Every philosopher talks about the power of energy. Since the connection between the parent and the child is naturally very strong, the energy flow between them is as though they were Siamese twins, sharing one heart and one brain. Quite simply, the parent's thoughts become part of the child's, even if the child is unconscious and even if the child is too young to be able to interpret and understand the facts. The life force can function and fight for health much better when positively charged. If the child has temporarily lost it, it is in our power to recharge his power. A good thought, a smile, a soft touch, a loving voice, a "beautiful ride on the rainbow" of imagination and visualization, and allowing no doubt or fear near the child, helps more than 10 truckloads of medications.

Self-fulfilling prophecy children must know

Thoughts become things, make them good

When Anna became very ill, she was surprised as she realized how she was the creator of her disease. The old saying always prompts us: "Don't say it or it will come to you," or "Beware of what you wish for, you may get it," or "Say it out loud so God will hear you." The concept of praying to God and asking him for something or wish, should be taught to our children. It is basically the same as the law of attraction, though wish lists have to do with birthdays, or holidays. Plant that seed of awareness into your children's minds. It may sound a bit odd to be written by such an experienced naturopathic doctor but it is true and worth considering as a tool for positive development of your children. When we meditate or sit in church in the pew, or kneel down to pray, or stand in front of the Torah, we are submissive to the higher power for our wishes to come true.

Children have even more power to do so, because their minds are still open to their imagination and they are not skeptical or cynical yet. Children have no doubt that there is a higher power and that it is their parent or guardian. Many of us practice our religion, some of us surround ourselves with all kinds of "guardian angels," sacred places, sacred ornaments and we may not like to compare it to a "child's imagination" but it is so. We need the belief that there is help, that there is luck, that there is mercy and love. We call it "hope", "faith", "God", "universe" "light", "light at the end of the tunnel", "miracles", "good energy", "crystals", "angels", "pixies", "trolls", "Yod", etc. No matter what we call it, we all share in this belief of a higher power.

The children are drawn into these beliefs as if they are just a given fact of life, and that is their biggest asset. All we need to do is help the children to keep these little "helpers" and make them work for them. When a child learns to be positive that this little angel or even rock will help him get out of trouble, he will adopt a lifelong friend. What the child will actually get is the ability to possess the trust and love in him. We do not need any fancy toys to be happy or healthy. We need our little friend who will always answer our prayers. Like little Alice, who believed that there was a little friend in her that was doing anything he could to help her heal. Like Omrie, when she was sitting in the bathtub and could envision herself in the open fields with these beautiful horses and flowers. Today, Omrie is 14 years old and she says, "I will never forget that bath." She also realized that the power of goodness, health, love, courage and life is in her. All she needs to do is just close her eyes - and there it is.

When a child learns the power of visualization, meditation, or prayer, it will easily understand that the same power, if used in a negative way, may bring the unwanted thoughts into his reality. It is important to be constructive and positive in our thinking. When I talked about the media and its negativity, I suggested that violence would attract violence for the child. The violence in the TV games, movies and news are understood by the kids as a way of handling problems. That is not by any means a fertile ground for a healthy development of children's mind and imagination. Children tend to be copycat and some of them are so drawn into their imagination that they harm others and themselves. Just as our imagination can heal and support us, negative imaginings do the same, but in a destructive way. The universe does not discriminate between good and bad thoughts; this is up to us. Like attracts like. As so many times we say: "similar attracts similar", "it takes one to know one", "like magnetizes like." If a child decides to "punish" his mother and become sick, it will get sick. Our obligation is to help our kids to learn to channel their own thoughts in a constructive passage. If the child learns to express his or her feelings, talk about them, draw them or dance them and the parents are open to listen and explain, or respond in a constructive way, the child will never become destructive, neither in his thoughts nor in his actions. If the child has constantly been pushed away and not listened to, it will internalize the thoughts, anger, grief, disappointment and fear, and may become very destructive, either towards himself, or towards anyone or anything in his daily life.

When Anna had no listeners and no sympathy it only added to her homesickness. She missed her family and friends overseas; she could not wait to grow up and actually dreamed of literally flying back home.

This was when she chose death. She wrote in her diary and manifested her dreams. She fulfilled her self-prophecy. When she realized what she had done, it was too late because it was her decision to put an end to her suffering, and she could not find the "key" to reverse the process. The self-fulfilling prophecy is extremely powerful and kids must learn it from early on for their protection. We must teach them the secret of only good thoughts for themselves. They will eventually lead them to their goals and make their dreams come true. However, instead of warning them how bad it could get, which could implant unnecessary and unwanted ideas in their mind, the best way would be to approach it only through a positive way. We want to teach our children the power in ourselves to manifest everything wonderful we wish for. Everything that is good for us of course.

Does it sound weird to you teaching your children the power of their own thoughts and wishes? When my children were very young and asked me to teach them astrology, my husband insisted, "Do not plant this nonsense in their minds." I believed then, and still do, that astrology is a natural, positive and wonderful asset for any child to be introduced to. To learn and understand the interconnection and influence of other planets upon our planet. To understand the energy exchange between planets and how they reflect on our planet and our own life. I would rather introduce them to this ancient empirical knowledge than to the TV. I prefer to see the belief in the mighty powers of the universe and positive thinking being fostered at home, than time spent under the disruptive influence of the media, and the violent electronic games. I would rather see the child's imagination encouraged towards the positive, than the way the terrorists raise innocent young children to seek death and murder in the name of God. Only through cultivating our children's positive assets of their personal beliefs and imagination will the future generation stop the insanity our world is experiencing now. Our children, with their guided positive attitude will shake off the madness and destruction, the greed and corruption, and will create a completely new life and a health-seeking world. God bless them for that. God bless you parents for contributing to that effort. This is basically what we had in mind when we brought our children into this world. We brought them up with the prayer that they would see a better world than what the present situation is.

Many of us try to grasp quantum physics and are intimidated by it. We had learned since childhood that when something falls, it simply falls down and not up. This is true. However, the truth is that everything is energy, and that everything we do is energy, and everything we wish for is energy. Moreover, whatever we think is energy and will manifest into matter that is also energy.

Children have a much easier time grasping these concepts and it is very strengthening and comforting to them. I strongly believe that through a simple little rock a child may learn to find its connection with his inner power, or God and that connection is worth a million doses of Ritalin.

Alon was a very normal boy but with many behavioral difficulties. The non-stop scolding and discipline was all he heard throughout. He was very angry with the people around him who criticized his behavior which only worsened things and created social problems in school as well. Neighbors complained about his intimidating behavior and the school system strongly pushed for medical treatments to alter his behavior and lessen his emotional aggressive behavior.

His mother bravely refused to put her son on any medication and went to seek advice other than medicine. I suggested giving him a little rock like I had given to my own grandchildren, for his birthday with a tiny key. I explained to Alon to hold the rock between his two hands every night before he goes to bed and thank God. He was supposed to thank God for at least three good things he experienced that day. After a week he returned and said; "I noticed how joyous life has been on a daily basis and how I overlooked them - for my thoughts of anger that occupied my mind". Then I asked him to list four good things he had done that day, also. And for the tiny key; the key was for when "you feel the need to talk to God, close your eyes, and knock on the imaginary door that leads to God, and when you hear "Come in," open the door with this tiny key and find that god has all the time you need, and boundless love just for you."

Needless to say, the mother was a little apprehensive and probably doubted my sanity. It did not take more than a couple of days before the child was unrecognizable. His behavior at home, in school and in his neighborhood changed so significantly that the teacher asked the mother what Alon was taking. She simply smiled and said: "Yael showed him the way to him and God with a small rock and a tiny key."

Alon followed the "instructions" religiously every night and told me about his magnificent results.

To help our children we need to just tune into the nature of the child. The power of imagination can be harnessed for the best outcomes. It is a gift your child will never lose, never forget, and benefit for the rest of his life. In addition - it is not addictive.

A child will never outgrow this gift, and it never wears out. Even if the child were to lose the rock, it will always stay with him by the power of imagination.

Supporting the child in his imagination and helping him channel his thoughts in a constructive way, may make the difference for a healthier generation and a healthier nation and most likely even a better world. It is in our power to make the change. It is easy, fun, rewarding and long lasting. No need for a doctor to "prescribe" this medication and no need to be licensed for it. All you need is to go to your child's room, tuck him into his bed and tell him how you would like him to

"Join you" on the ride to a better place. How you would like to give him this precious little rock to connect to eternity and to God, and to all that is good. It is simple and your child will treasure it and keep it forever. Your child will feel elated like never before. They do not need to dress up for church, or synagogue, for that connection with the higher power. They do not need to fear God, just love and be thankful.

Children must learn from all their prayer to pray only for their higher best, and never for any destructive wish.

Dreams

Dreams are invaluable in finding the cause of any problem a child may have. Dreams actually reveal to us, in various snapshots or videos, which are filed away in the child's inner archive. All of the fears, sorrows, disappointments, and anxieties the child is unable to address in its waking hours, come alive in his dreams. When children are unduly restless just prior to their normal bedtime, it may be a good idea to look into their dreams and see if there is a culprit. Spend a little time trying to discover what makes bedtime unpleasant. When your child describes his dreams, consider yourself a lucky parent. Because your child actually opens an important little window for you to peek into his innermost world.

This is a real treasure for any therapist who knows the importance and significance of the correlation between the soul, emotions, mind and body. So, next time when your child is trying to describe his dream to you do not just comfort the child, and say, "Oh, dear, it's just a dream." But better sit down and listen attentively until the child has fully explained his thoughts, and if you like, take some notes. Ask yourself questions and consider what may be at the center of your child's dreams: "What were we talking about today?" "What did the child eat or drink today?" What did he experience that troubled him?" These are just a few examples of the many things you like to consider when a child is having unsettling dreams. For the child who is pre-verbal, offer some paper and crayons, and ask the child to draw you a picture of its dream. Keep in mind that children are more sensitive than most adults are, and therefore may have much more meaningful dreams than we do.

As many other reputable health practitioners have discovered, I have often been lucky enough to find the clue to a child's health problem in his or her dreams. No wonder dreams are considered the porthole to the hidden secrets of the soul. It is revealing the whole picture with details and revelations the child could never fully capture in his waking moments.

At times, when very bad dreams come up I suggest serving dinner earlier, making absolutely sure that no fat and meat are on the menu. If your child continues to complain of nightmares, switch the meals between lunch and dinner. The liver functions between 4 a.m. and 6 p.m., thus anything the child eats after 6 p.m. just sits in his stomach undigested until morning. This creates pressure on the pit of the stomach, where the Vagus nerve and main artery run through to the abdomen. This nerve is the connecting nerve between the academic brain and the parasympathetic system like, heart, lungs and stomach. It is also named the Pneumogastric nerve, since it travels through the lungs and the stomach, ending in the colon. Think of the Latin root of the word, 'Vagus', meaning literally "to wander". Knowing this bit of biology will help you to better understand the importance of not allowing late night eating to interfere with this nerve, as it is so interwoven through our whole system.

Giggling Dr. Green

When the heavy weight of a full stomach presses on these vessels, the oxygen supply suffers and the brain produces these frightening images, causing it to wake up and gasp for air and thrash about. However, dreams are not necessarily just nightmares. Dreams can certainly also be very pleasant, offering us a privileged glimpse into the child's inner world of fanciful beauty. For many years, I have used children's vibrant dreams as keys to unlock the mysteries behind their suffering and complaints.

Please, also make absolutely certain that the child is not exposed to any violent movies or news on TV, especially before bedtime.

A good conversation, soft, classic music, a pleasant time of storytelling or reading and a light meal could be an easy but very effective solution to a child's bad dreams.

Another way to address dreams with children is to encourage them to act out their dreams and the characters in them with puppets. As the child gives a daytime face to his nighttime fears, he will often be able to work through the anguish disturbing his sleep. This is a wonderful way to conquer the 'monsters' and make them less threatening.

As a grown up, I began experiencing recurring dreams involving huge lions and tigers in front of every door of my home. They frightened me until I finally realized they must represent a message to me, but my conscience did not know what it was. When I told my friend about it, she was amused, but offered no guidance. However, just speaking to her helped me understand that these dreams told me something about my fear of freedom. But, how could it be? I have always been the "queen of freedom" and this has always been my most important goal. Freedom of speech, freedom of thought, freedom for the soul, mind, body. Any sports or recreational activity had to be outdoors, I would feel too confined indoors. So, why would I fear freedom? Yet, if the message my subconscious mind was giving me was my fear of freedom, something clearly was not adding up and needed further thought. Very often, dreams will not make sense or else they would not need to come in disguises and symbols, and we would be able to express our concerns and worries easily in words.

It took me a long time to figure out the puzzle my dreams had created. When I recovered fully from my fears, I had the same dream, yet, this time the huge lions and tigers shrunk into little puppies and were on a leash in the back seat of my car. So it was the same dream, but with a completely different feeling and meaning.

Giggling Dr. Green

We all dream, and we should appreciate our dreams as a very important and relevant part of our life and our total well-being. Our children can learn to use their dreams and help us heal their own illnesses, anxieties, and diseases. If a small child learns how to accept and deal with his own dreams, or learns to appreciate them as an important message from the inner self, he or she will grow up to be a well-adjusted adult, with far less hidden fears and apprehensions. Another way to help your child to deal with his dreams is by sharing your own dreams and being honest in discussing them with your child. It helps children to cope with their fears, anxieties and imaginations when they realize how we are like them, still dreaming as if we were little children as well.

The beauty in the visualization technique is the tools we develop to help create our own dreams and to gain the power to create the reality that suits our needs. In this same way, dreams work for us as long as we regard and respect them as a telescope into the soul. Dreams are just a way to help us create reality while we are sleeping.

Since we know how the universe grows from a seed, so is our life. If we help our child to plant the seed, the child will be able to create the reality growing from that seed. In the dreams, we learn to see what is preventing or frightening the child away from pursuing the big dream, the dream of growing up strong in body, soul and mind

Traveling with children

As I already mentioned in the beginning of this book, when I'm asked if I take medications on my trips I say; I take my hands with me. That is my most valuable medicine if you will.

Since my children were little babies, I would grab their feet when they were sick and give them a thorough reflexology treatment. It was funny how they would lay down and push their little feet to me when they were feeling a little sick. Shay was my best "little client." He really hated to be sick and instead of wanting to be pampered and spoiled always was very eager to get well as soon as possible. He would never stay in bed more than absolutely necessary. The children knew they could feel better after just one treatment and never thought anything else could help as much.

Reflexology is a very natural healing art and can be easily learned by everyone. Even little children love to do it to their siblings and parents. Reflexology is based upon the idea of relaxation, like acupuncture - through the release of the natural endorphins into the blood, and by the stimulation of the lymphatic circulation. We all know by now that the minute the lymphatic fluid starts moving, the pain lifts, the cramps disappear and the self-healing mechanism starts to kick in.

Shay's graduation party from daycare took place when he developed a high fever, and was unable to attend the celebration. These fevers of Shay's always seemed to occur at the most inconvenient moments. The fastest remedy I had at hand - were my hands. I took his small feet in my hands, and within just 10 minutes of treatment Shay was up and running to join the party. I never used medications for our children, even when we had to face minor illnesses at terribly inconvenient times and places such as on a plane or bus or at a hotel. We just used what we had - our hands and their feet, or spine, or hands, as the case may be. Over the years, I have taught this technique throughout the world, and I have gotten amazing feedback from those who continue to swear by it to this day.

When Omrie was just 3 years old, she would come with a little towel and a jar of lotion and would give me a very pleasant and soothing little treatment with her little hands. It is hard to believe how even those little, soft, light hands with almost insignificant pressure could make one feel so much better, even though it was coming from a young child. I urge every parent to take a little course for an overall basic idea of reflexology, and have it at hand, literally, at all times. When you know how to apply it, you free yourself of any fear of not having the proper medications. You do not need a doctor; your hands are the doctor!

In Estes Park, Colorado, Tal said to me; "Mom, look at those people there!" He pointed his finger to a small group of people surrounding an elderly woman, as she was turning very pale. It was clear that she was feeling very bad and weak. They seemed to be contemplating what to do, and how best to help her.

I stepped up to the woman and said, "May I please try to help you?" She looked at me and said weakly, "But I can't take any medication." That is quite alright I smiled, I don't have any. All I need is your hands for a moment with your permission, of course." She answered me with a very pale, little weak smile and offered me her hands. It took just a few minutes of reflexology treatment for her color to come back and she began to feel better.

She was so very grateful, and I felt thankful to have had my little "portable" medicine kit with me wherever I am. Since I see the necessity and benefit of this basic knowledge, I created a very thorough reflexology course on DVD, so that everyone will be able to learn the basics at home. Although it is mandatory in many states in America to have 500 hours of massage school in order to be licensed to use reflexology, I still think that it is everyone's right, and I feel it is our responsibility to help every parent and family member to learn any available way to help other family members heal, with or without the rules and regulations. I agree that we cannot treat clients and get paid for the reflexology basics, but, I also agree that it is a very natural way to help each other in every home and every family, like Shiatsu, Yoga, Reiki, Hands on, Crystals, Juicing, Conversation, Wet towels, etc.

These are my suggestions, offered to you, for your family's good health. Please do not take this book as though it were the inspired word of God, and do not complain or become discouraged if you do not achieve immediate results. It takes time to learn and you will need to be devoted in your home practices. After all, every art of healing, and every medical application, is just a search, a suggestion to try. The idea behind it all is that these are tools for natural health that exist just for us, and it is something that cannot be regulated by a government office, nor taxed or franchised.

Virtues - top priority

The mandatory bible classes in every school in Israel are too many children a thorn, as they had been for my children. The kids thought it was the most boring class ever and often wondered aloud, "Who needs all this anyway?" They wondered why the bible lessons have not been removed from our schools like in many countries where religion has been completely removed from the school system. I agree that in a melting pot like America, where so many different cultures and ethnicities gather in one classroom, it would be totally out of line to teach just one religion. I believe in freedom of religion and the freedom not to be forced to participate in it as well. Israel is also a melting pot but officially promotes the Jewish faith, especially following the devastating Holocaust that forced the Jewish people to reclaim their historical right of the one place on the planet where they will never be persecuted or considered, strange minority ever again. All the wars Israel has fought the past 60 years are due to this one fact. A nation that believes in the Bible needs a piece of land that can be called home. This is the only explanation for the Bible studies in Israel's schools, in times when there are not many other religious teachings in public classrooms anymore.

However, by removing religion out of the schools, we removed a great deal of important respect and values teachings from the classrooms. Sadly, we find ever more parents, teachers, schools, and even governments putting the emphasis on teaching professional and financial success before values. If values are not our first priority in life, our society, community, families and even ourselves, we lose the true essence of being human. It is sad how the students are tested for reading

Giggling Dr. Green

and writing and math skills, yet not asked even one question about values. Children who attend (most, but not all) religious ceremonial congregations are usually exposed to the basic values and respect for God. The Ten Commandments are just the tip of the iceberg in a long list of important values for every person. It must be repeated daily, consistently so children are drawn to the important values instead of pushing them away. I am quoting the Bible nearly every day when talking with my students, children, friends or clients, since I went to the same schools in Israel, and though I am not practicing the Jewish religion, the wisdom I absorbed from the bible are invaluable and worthy of passing on.

Gail did not stop talking about how orthodox religious they were and desperately she and her husband would do anything, truly anything, to have a child. After a course of treatments, Gail finally conceived and gave birth to a healthy beautiful boy. When she returned to my office, I heard how much she loved her baby. However, the baby had a few problems, and was not as she would have really liked it to be. It had dark hair and dark eyes, instead of blue eyes and blond hair.

Gail as well as her husband had dark hair and dark eyes.

Well, I said, you are so religious yet, never satisfied. Even God cannot please you. You so desperately prayed for a child, and now, you got it, and instead of being grateful for it and its health, you complain about hair and eye color. Being a very religious woman, she was willing to accept my comments when I said; you know that God created us in his own image, as the Bible says. That means: if you doubt the perfection of your child, you doubt God. If you're so religious, how can you doubt God? Where is the adage, who is the rich, the one is grateful for what he has. These are values to consider and teach children, as they prevent greed and jealousy and dishonesty.

She agreed since she realized that she does not appreciate herself. It would be great had Gail taught her children to be grateful for everything, which is part of the important values. She still complains about her 7-year-old boy who is "not good enough." This is exactly my point. If the boy is "not good enough," to whom does she compare him? Will the boy then learn to be satisfied and be grateful for who he is? Will this boy learn to appreciate others for who they are? On the other hand, will he be like his mother who is not happy and never satisfied even with her child's physical looks? Is it because others are blond with blue eyes, and she has to have what others have, because what she has is never good enough? This is a recipe for never-ending frustration and empty feeling. It is a recipe for depression and jealousy. It is at the core of poor health and social difficulties. When children grow up getting everything and anything they wish for and imagine, they get overwhelmed and do not appreciate the small things. Values are not about what we have and what we want. Values are about what we need to be grateful for and what good we can do for someone less fortunate, or just because we want to share well with others. Values are also the ability to accept others for who they are, regardless of their looks, hair and eye color, clothes, their car, or their economic status. Values are the ability and desire to be humble and modest. Values are the understanding that there must always be enough of everything, not just for us, but for others as well.

Virtues to me are far from being, dressed up all fancy and trying to make a good impression on others. Having to put up false facade and manners, yet still being very polite and considerate because we want others to think as if we have values - is wrong. Every person has a sensitive beating heart in his chest like our own heart. Every person has a loving mother who worries about him or her. If it were not for our own ego, we would let our hearts communicate between ourselves and leave the ego out of our relationships, meaning that success is very positive, provided we improve ourselves, but is negative if we want to beat our friends and prove they are less than we are. I realize that it is not the way reality is when our children grow up into the competitive world. However, think about how synchronicity works. Don't you want the world to be a better place for your children? Don't you wish that when your child grows up, the crime rate would drop so that you will not have to worry about your child ever being hurt by a stray bullet? Don't you pray that when your child grows up, it won't necessarily be Mr. Success, but just be happy, generally accepted, and won't feel like a failure? Wouldn't you like to see the drug addiction rate drop and people being kinder and more helpful to each other? It is not utopia; it is possible. Consider this; if one million mothers and fathers would read this book, or similar and would adopt this idea, they would raise their children by these values. In addition, let us imagine that each parent has three to five kids at home; each child has cousins, nieces and friends that would happily adopt these values as well. Millions of people could adopt the same values being number one on their priorities list. This could change the world in a matter of just one generation. You can make a difference and contribute to a better world for your kids and their friends. See how good, kind, and sacrificing and considerate people were on and after 9/11 in New York, and even all over the United States? See how many good, kind and helpful people turned out to help when Katrina hit New Orleans? I feel sorry for those looters who gave in to their weaker natures. However, there were thousands and probably millions of people who found the very best values in themselves and put their own comfort and lives aside for the sake of others, strangers. This just indicates that people have the values, compassion, and kindness in them. My question is only, why are people so good, kind and helpful under the worst circumstances but do not practice it in their daily lives? I believe that ingraining the values in our children, daily, we can change the world for your children into a better place. I strongly believe that children are so happy to be good, to help, share and love. All they need is consistent reminders, guidance, raising the bar of values a little higher every once in a while, appreciation and recognition. When children embrace the values we teach, it makes them ready to take that goodness into the world.

When you instill virtues in your children, not only will you be very proud of your child when time comes, but you will have fewer arguments and disagreements with your child. You will also be treated with respect, care, appreciation, consideration, compassion and love when you get older and are not as strong and self-sufficient any more. At times when you may need your grown up child to be at your side. You may also take comfort in knowing your child is happy with his or her family, job, and home, even if it may be just a small apartment. That will keep your child stress-free, happy, grateful, and therefore - most importantly- healthy. The grandkids will get the same upbringing and your family will be a healthy, harmonious and happy one. Like it says: "Love your neighbor like you love yourself".

Being grateful for our health, for who we are, for the privilege to get up in the morning and see the light, for the modest and simple food to eat and share, and for the roof on our head. To be appreciative of the lesson the universe allows us to learn and the opportunity to be kind, respectful and helpful to our world - Values to keep close to heart.

It is our duty and privilege to give this precious, indispensable gift of life to our children. Do not wait for any kindergarten nurse or teacher to do it for you. Just do it, daily and you will reap the fruit as your children grow up.

Teach your child this saying to be repeated every morning and every evening:

"Keep an attitude of gratitude."

Rob was about to celebrate his 10th birthday. He called his grandmother and said to her, "I need $800 for my new bike. When are you going to give me the money?" The wise grandmother was determined to teach her demanding grandson a little lesson in gratitude. She took a nice polished river rock, washed it and put it in a nice jewelry box. To the box, she added this little letter: "Dear Rob, since I love you so much, I am delighted to send you this beautiful magic rock. It is so beautiful because for many years the pounding water buffed the edges of the rock, polished and shined it. It took many years, a lot of water, and the power of a stream to shape this beautiful rock. I believe this rock could have been there even 300 years ago or perhaps even longer. The rock will help you to receive all you wish. There is just one condition to it: You must hold this rock in both hands every night before you go to sleep, and thank God, for at least three good things that happened to you today. Then you must thank God for at least three good things you do have in your life. In addition, the third thing you must do for the rock to work for you is; you must tell God at least four good things you have done today. I think that in the next three weeks, if you do it every day, you will see how all your wishes start to come true."

Rob received the little gift his grandmother sent him and said to her, "Thank you. I am very excited to start using this magic rock. I am so happy to receive your precious gift." (His response was a big surprise to his grandmother, because everyone around predicted that he would toss it and be very angry at her).

That night, his mom had to read him the "magic rock instructions" since he could not read his grandmother's handwriting very well.

This was that grandmother's way to "heal" Rob's lack of his poor manners and his demanding attitude, teach him gratitude and appreciation, and make him meditate each night on all the good he has in his life. Rob was very anxious to find four good things he could do every day, so he will be able to share with God his contribution to the world around him.

In such very simple ways, every child can develop an attitude of gratitude and grow up happier and healthier.

The most important way to teach our kids values and gratitude is by personal example. If we make it a priority in our life to be grateful and helpful to the world around us, our children will imitate us. If we will try to teach them values we do not honor, it will seem as hollow to them as an empty well.

This is a true example of how we do not give out the right message if we do not live the values we teach our children. I was sitting with a friend's child in their living room when the father was telling his son how bad it is to lie. How important it is to always say the truth, as suddenly the phone rings. The child picks up the phone and on the other end the voice asks for his dad. He held the phone down and said to his father: "Daddy, this man wants to talk to you", "Just tell him I am not home", the father answered. I wonder if this was the proper example of how not to lie.

I believe

I believe that every child is born with the basic right for good health, freedom, protection and justice.

I believe that every child has the right to be protected, even from the government if the rules and regulations are proven to be harmful and dangerous with a transparent source of information for us to make the educated choice for our child's utmost best.

I believe that scientific research and the true practice of health are completely different entities that do not work in unison. Science is knowledge accumulated through research, yet the manifestation of the knowledge is not used by the so-called "health providers" due quite simply to greed.

With all due respect to science, I believe that centuries of experience are a more reliable testimony than the ever-changing claims of modern science. I believe that by looking around, we see how we can help save the planet for our children, but there is a flipside to this: We must also look around and see how to save our children for the planet. All I brought here in this book are recommendations from the ancient healing arts, augmented and bolstered by my relatively short experience as a natural healer as well. I do not offer you any scientific approach to health, I make no suggestions for any type of medications, and would like my readers to acknowledge that I do not mean for this book to be used as a medical book. I believe that homeopathy, reflexology, PEMF, water applications, juicing and all the many other natural approaches though are just suggestions - are still the best healing methods the human kind developed and experienced throughout centuries; there are no mandates or specific recipes for success in this book. I have gathered here a collection of many different cultures' healing arts. However, since these are the methods I have been using for my own family, for myself, and for clients throughout the world for over 4 decades, I am convinced that they are the best way to achieve sustainable and long lasting health. These applications and treatments are noninvasive, harmless ideas for promoting health and well-being for our children and ourselves. It is your own responsibility when using any or all these methods, to remember, in case of life or death - seek medical attention without delay. Countless families around the globe have chosen the path I have shown here in this book, and have thanked me for their very lives. It takes a leap of faith in order to stop struggling with the side effects of the pills, powders and madness imposed by the MEGA Force, but you will never look back once you have experienced a drug free existence.

Giggling Dr. Green

I find animal research irrelevant, because people are not to be compared and measured by the same indicators as mice.

In turn I ask if this research had ever heard a mouse, or guinea pig complain about their stressful, abusive marriage, or a home foreclosure or her children's behavior disorders. If we take only the physical information and observations from any other creature, or even from a different person, we will never get any accurate results and answers to the individual problem.

I believe and pray that it will not be very long before the medical establishment finally steps back to the point before it started dividing the human body into different parts, and will appreciate and acknowledge the whole human being again, for true and successful medical help. I pray that people will be treated individually and not as case numbers. I have no answers for diseases by their labels and names, because I do not believe in diseases. I believe in Dis-Ease and in looking for the message in every disease.

I believe that every disease is the way our life force draws our attention when threatened and in distress. I believe that under any circumstances the cause and reason should be addressed as they may be very different from the cause and reason any mouse rat or guinea pig would possibly have. Therefore, the conclusions and treatments should be, according to my logic, very different from those we would suggest for a mouse or a guinea pig. I believe that there is not even one disease that can be addressed by physical and chemical treatments alone. We have to treat the wholeness.

I pray that labs will be just a last resort and that the doctors will take more time to see the person, why and where the problem manifests in that person's body.

I believe and pray that children will not be "shot" any more for their very "doubtful" and deceptive "health benefit", but will grow up with the right to develop a healthy immune system sustaining them in a healthy, fulfilling life.

I believe that this book is just one teardrop in an ocean of cries to stop the victimization of our children by the mandatory criminal health services, the ones that only exist to keep the mad cycle of the healthcare industry going.

Thank you for working your way through this book, and I hope each of you will find some help in it.

Yours in good health

Yael Shany

Giggling Dr. Green

Giggling Dr. Green

www.ingramcontent.com/pod-product-compliance
Lightning Source LLC
Chambersburg PA
CBHW061627250726

48659CB00004B/1113